INTERNATIONAL PSYCHOTHERAPY

INTERNATIONAL PSYCHOTHERAPY

Theories, Research, and Cross-Cultural Implications

EDITED BY
Lynn Simek-Downing

PRAEGER

New York
Westport, Connecticut
London

The International Conference on Psychotherapy held in Bogotá, Colombia, in 1983 was subsidized by the Universidad de los Andes. The papers from the conference were collected by Dr. Augusto Perez-Gomez and Dr. Fernando Barrera.

Copyright Acknowledgments

Portions of Chapter 3 are reprinted with permission of Guilford Press from P. L. Wachtel, *Action and Insight* (New York: Guilford, 1987).

Chapter 4 is reprinted with permission of the American Association for Counseling and Development, which published it under the same title in *Counseling and Values,* April 1985, pp. 99-116.

Chapter 5 is reprinted with permission of Dow Jones–Irwin from M. J. Lambert, ed., *Psychotherapy and Patient Relationships* (Homewood, Ill.: Dow Jones-Irwin, 1983), pp. 85-125.

Chapter 8 is reprinted with permission from "Eclecticism and Integration in Psychotherapy," Sol Garfield, *Behavior Therapy,* vol. 13 (1982): 610-23. Copyright 1982 by the Association for Advancement of Behavior Therapy. Reprinted by permission of the publisher and author.

Portions of Chapter 11 are reprinted with permission of Guilford Press from L. S. Greenberg and W. M. Pinsof, eds., *The Psychotherapeutic Process: A Research Handbook* (New York: Guilford Press, 1986).

A portion of Chapter 13 is reprinted with permission of *Family Medicine* from L. Simek-Downing and M. Quirk, "Videotape Analyses of Medical Students' Interviewing Skills," *Family Medicine* 17, no. 2 (March–April 1985): 57-60.

Library of Congress Cataloging-in-Publication Data

International psychotherapy : theories, research, and cross-cultural
implications / edited by Lynn Simek-Downing.
p. cm.
Includes index.
ISBN 0-275-93096-3 (alk. paper)
1. Psychiatry, Transcultural. I. Simek-Downing, Lynn.
RC455.4.E8167 1989
150—dc19 88-26578

Library of Congress Catalog Card Number: 88-26578
ISBN: 0-275-93096-3

First published in 1989

Praeger Publishers, One Madison Avenue, New York, NY 10010
A division of Greenwood Press, Inc.

Printed in the United States of America

The paper used in this book complies with the Permanent Paper Standard issued by the National Information Standards Organization (Z39.48—1984).

10 9 8 7 6 5 4 3 2 1

This book is dedicated with love to Drew and Lindsay.

A very special thanks to Deborah LeBreton for her work and support in text preparation.

Contents

Preface

This book originated with the idea that the many people of the world who practice in the art of psychotherapy in various capacities should be brought together in one arena. The art and science of helping is conducted in all languages and cultures of the world, and yet distinct differences are seen in these practices that are relative to the people within each culture. The cultural and political context of psychotherapy in developing nations has a different nature than it does in technologically advanced societies, and even more distinct differences emerge between the need for and the process of psychotherapy in capitalist versus socialist versus communist nations. While the cultural and political variants seem to further isolate and separate nations, the need for psychotherapy, to help people, remains the same throughout the world. People of all nations and political beliefs experience grief, loss, pain, difficulties in life, and trauma. We are all different and we are all the same.

The first convergence of a multinational assembly of people working in the field of psychotherapy happened at the International Conference on Psychotherapy held in Bogotá, Colombia, in 1983. Many nations and four continents were represented, and papers and workshops were given by scholars on all aspects of psychotherapeutic practice, research, and theoretical models. The chapters in this book are representative of the work of some of the presenters from this conference.

I have divided the book into three sections to represent three themes that emerge in issues of cross-cultural considerations of psychotherapy: social implications, theories, and research. In each section, authors are represented from different cultures and countries. The authors are professors of psychology or psychotherapy from around the world and present divergent viewpoints. Many of them refer to and critique each others' work in the included chapters. The discussions are often lively and entail a profound knowledge of one anothers' work although separated by oceans and continents.

The time has come in the developing science and art of psychotherapy to join with our fellows and create a new state of the art that goes beyond individual differences and lends itself to the pursuit of cultural understanding and wisdom that will more completely serve the needs of the people in the global village. A uniting of our understanding of people, both within their cultural context and as people of the world, can further the practice of psychotherapy by sharing resources, knowledge, understanding, and wisdom. This book is a beginning on that path of sharing. This work is dedicated to the healing and helping of the people of all the nations of the world. May we work toward a common goal.

Introduction: Converging Themes in Psychotherapy

Michael J. Mahoney

In 1983 I was given the opportunity to make some brief comments on the significance of the International Conference on Psychotherapy and its potential role in the further refinement of our understanding and facilitation of human development. To my regret, I could not attend the conference in person. Many of the participants were respected friends and colleagues, and the conference was a historic event in the evolution of the art, science, and profession of psychotherapy. The field owes a debt of gratitude to Augusto Perez Gomez and his colleagues for having initiated and actualized such a progressive and stimulating encounter among the divergent approaches.

Of the major issues and themes that are central to the refinement of this area, four strike me as the most provocative for this discussion.

First, to what extent do our tacit models of human nature limit, distort, or otherwise influence our more explicit models of psychotherapy and general change processes? This is obviously a "metaquestion", but it is one of the most important ones we can pose. Humanistic psychologists, for example, have a clearly different model of human nature than do orthodox psychoanalysts and behavioral modifiers. How do these models affect the therapist's conceptualization and conduct of that fascinating and humbling human enterprise we term "psychotherapy"?

Second, what are the range and limits of human malleability? The human organism is clearly a paradox of infinite options within, to borrow

Hayek's phrase, discernible "contexts of constraint." For almost a century now, we have realized how difficult it is for many individuals to produce meaningful and enduring changes in some patterns of their lives. The continuing search for the parameters of malleability is an important one, but it pales before the more fundamental question of how much the human nervous system can change and how we, as clinical scientists, can meaningfully identify and measure the most important aspects of that change.

Third, what are the basic processes involved in human change? This deceptively simple question will probably consume our interest for some time. It is clear that our traditional theories have yet to offer much more than crude descriptions of selected regularities in human change. We still know very little, for example, about the synergistic roles of emotional arousal, behavioral activation, and the dynamic reciprocity of cognitive assimilation and accommodation.

And fourth, do the questions emanating from this conference reflect upon our current understanding and, more importantly, our strategies for studying human experience and life counseling? More specifically, what do our questions tell us about our basic assumptions and the directions toward which we seem to be moving?

In other words, the following are the four fundamental questions in our inquiry:

(1) How do our tacit models of human nature influence our theories and therapies?
(2) What are the constraints upon human change?
(3) What are the basic processes of that change?
(4) What are our basic assumptions and methods of inquiry?

It is, of course, much easier to pose questions than to answer them. But, we should remember that the depth of our understanding is more often reflected in the quality of our questions than in that of our answers.

A brief quotation will convey the spirit of our quest in a more eloquent fashion. These words were written by Bertrand Russell in his autobiography, late in his life as he reflected upon his own intellectual and humanitarian ventures. They were published as the prologue to his autobiography:

> Three passions, simple but overwhelmingly strong, have governed my life: the longing for love, the search for knowledge, and unbearable pity of the suffering of mankind. These passions like great winds, have blown me hither and thither, in a wayward course, over a deep ocean of anguish, reaching the very verge of despair. I have sought love, first, because it brings ecstasy--ecstasy so great that I would often have sacrificed all the rest of life for a few hours of this joy. I have sought it, next, because it relieves loneliness--that terrible loneliness in which one shivering consciousness looks over the realm of the world into the cold unfathomable lifeless abyss. I have sought it, finally, because in the union of love I have seen, in a mystic miniature, the prefiguring vision of the heaven that saints and poets have imagined. This is what I sought, and though it might seem too good for human life, this is what--at least--I have found.
>
> With equal passion I have sought knowledge. I have wished to understand the hearts of men. I have wished to know why the stars shine. And I have tried to apprehend the Pythagorean power by which number holds sway above the flux. A little of this, but not much, I have achieved.
>
> Love and knowledge, so far as they were possible, led upward toward the heavens. But always pity brought me back to earth. Echoes of cries of pain reverberate in my heart. Children in famine, victims tortured by oppressors, helpless old people a hated burden to their sons, and the whole world of loneliness, poverty, and pain make a mockery of what human life should be. I long to alleviate the evil, but I cannot, and I too suffer.
>
> This has been my life. I have found it worth living, and would gladly live it again if the chances were offered me.[1]

May your experience enrich, deepen, and affirm our collective commitment to the nurturance of human development.

NOTE

1. *The Autobiography of Bertrand Russell*, (London: Allen & Unwin, 1967), Vol. 1, p. 13.

PART I

SOCIAL IMPLICATIONS OF PSYCHOTHERAPY

1

The Politics of Psychotherapy: Themes, Dilemmas, and Possibilities

Nick Heather

In addressing the topic of psychotherapy and politics, it is tempting to begin with a definition of the word. However, so many definitions are possible that to single out one of them might restrict the scope of this discussion in undesirable ways. Rather than attempt a formal definition, I shall merely point to the usage of the term I have in mind and some of its frequent connotations.

I am not concerned merely with the aspect of government or with the philosophies and programs of specific political parties, but with politics in a much wider sense. At a macro level, politics is the way in which societies are organized, how their resources are utilized, and how their material and cultural products are distributed. At the micro level, relationships between individual members of small groups, such as family units, are assumed, partly at least, to reflect relationships existing at higher levels of organization.

Also included in this kind of usage are the ideologies that may be found in a society. Again, "politics" is used in the most general sense, referring to the values and goals of life commonly accepted by members of a society and the justifications for existing social arrangements typically espoused by them. Finally, in virtue of the inclusion of "ideologies" in my terms of reference, I shall discuss the way the world, and particularly the world of human relationships, is experienced by individuals, insofar as this reflects objective relationships in society, in R. D. Laing's phrase, "the politics of experience."[1]

The use of "politics" and "ideologies" all refer to relationships of power and dominance among individuals and groups. This would include power relationships between societies as well as those within them.

THE RELEVANCE OF POLITICS

My intention in this chapter is to characterize the psychotherapeutic relationship as political, in the sense of politics just described. In literature devoted to the political context of psychotherapy, three related but clearly identifiable themes may be discovered, and I will discuss each in turn. But before doing so, it may be as well to give a general defense of the idea that political concerns are of relevance to psychotherapy and, in fact, demonstrate the folly of ignoring them. This defense will be necessary should anyone object that, reduced to its essentials, psychotherapy is simply a means of providing help for people in psychological distress, or "an interpersonal process designed to bring about modifications of feelings, cognition, attitudes and behavior which have proven troublesome to the person seeking help from a trained professional,"[2] or whatever other terms are preferred. By this argument, psychotherapy is independent of the type of society in which it occurs, and its success or failure is beyond the influence of political forces. Any attempt to drag politics into the discussion can only lead to confusion and retard the progress of psychotherapeutic methods. This might be an objection to the title of this chapter.

In a similar vein, it could be argued that the practice of medicine is essentially apolitical. People will become ill in any conceivable kind of society, and the task of medicine is simply to respond to this illness in the most efficient manner possible. Political considerations are at best irrelevant and at worst downright mischievous. In such a view, medical science and practice, and indeed basic and applied science in general, are purely logical, technical, and value free and must be carried on unhindered by moral and political constraints. This view of medicine, although extraordinarily naive, will provide an opportunity to illustrate by analogy the danger of omitting political considerations from discussions of psychotherapy.

The work of Thomas McKeown[3] has demonstrated clearly that the enormous improvements in health, as shown by the decline in mortality, in Britain and other developed nations over the last 300 years have been caused by the rapid reduction, followed by the virtual disappearance, of infectious diseases. However, the outstanding reasons for this reduction, McKeown goes on to show, do not lie in the wider or improved application of clinical medicine or in the accumulation of scientific knowledge regarding the pathological mechanisms and effective cures of the diseases in question. Instead, the reasons for the reductions lie in the vast social and economic changes that have taken place during this period. The causal irrelevance of medical interventions can be easily grasped from the fact that the decline in mortality preceded the widespread application of clinical methods and the discovery of specific remedies such as antibiotics. The revolution in health has been brought about by improvements in nutrition, water supply, housing, drainage, sewage disposal and the like, combined with a decrease in the rate of reproduction. The same set of factors also applies to the health of developing nations during this century, although here the separation of causal influences is more complex because environmental changes coincide with medical innovations. Many people, would regard as close to blasphemy, the suggestion that the greater length of their life expectation, compared with that of their recent ancestors, owes more to the growth of working-class power through the trade union movement than to the skill and dedication of the medical profession, and yet this is indeed the case.

The diseases mentioned by McKeown that were eradicated, leading to the decline in mortality, are all preventable diseases associated with poverty. However, the effects of poverty on health in advanced industrial societies have by no means disappeared, and poverty remains the single, most important factor in the probability of contracting a whole range of fatal and disabling diseases. In Britain, a country well known for its "socialist" system of medicine, there remain striking differences between socioeconomic classes with respect to all manner of indices of death and ill health. The evidence for this statement has been collected in the so-called Black Report,[4] which the British government, having failed to suppress, is trying to ignore. Thus political issues are still immediately relevant to the provision of health care within developed countries and are, of course, even more obviously applicable to international comparisons between rich and poor countries.[5]

Despite the continuing contribution of poverty

to the causes of disease, it is now commonly and correctly asserted that the major killers in advanced industrial societies--cancer, heart disease, and liver cirrhosis--are all diseases, not of poverty, but of affluence. Here, too, political considerations are immediately apparent. The need for governments to continue collecting huge revenues from taxes on cigarettes, alcohol, and other potentially harmful products, as well as to sustain the profits of the international companies which manufacture them, places the prevention of these diseases unequivocally in the political arena. For instance, it is now generally recognized by experts in the field of alcohol problems that the effectiveness of treatment services pales into insignificance compared with the potential impact of fiscal policies, including at the simplest level in the prices set on alcoholic beverages. However, the British government also suppressed the report of its own Central Policy Review Unit,[6] which put forward this argument.

While on the subject of diseases of affluence, one must not forget the contribution of industrial pollution to the increase in cancer and the reluctance of governments to enact or enforce legislation to reduce it. Finally, on the most general level, the stresses of living that are essential to the perpetuation of industrial societies are a further major contributor to modern forms of premature death.

All these are ways in which politics are relevant to the role of medicine in society. This demonstrates that political considerations can be shown to be relevant even where they may not appear to be. Each of the points made regarding the political context of medicine invites a parallel observation in the field of psychotherapy, and the fact that psychotherapy is practiced, more often than not, in a medical setting gives the analogy added force. Nevertheless, the relevance of politics to psychotherapy itself arises from more particular considerations, and to these I now turn.

Psychotherapy as a means of disguising the social and economic nature of human problems

Most laymen are surprised by the conclusion of McKeown's work regarding the environmental causes of infectious diseases, presumably because they have been told so often that modern improvements in health are due entirely to the achievements of medical science. There is an obvious advantage to the medical profession in this distortion, but it may also have a deeper ideological significance. By disguising the overriding importance of the political context of human health and disease with this mechanistic view of disease processes as involving a breakdown of functioning occurring inside individual persons, attention is deflected from the need to change the environment in the interest of healthier living.[7]

Exactly the same kind of charge can be made against psychotherapy and its theoretical relation to human problems. By locating the problem to be solved inside individual clients, psychotherapy disguises the need to change the social and economic conditions from which these problems arise. To substantiate this thesis, here, it is necessary to show that many problems the psychotherapist is confronted with do have socioeconomic origins.

As an example of a problem frequently dealt with by psychotherapists let us take depressions found in women. This has been the subject of an extensive, thorough, and methodologically sophisticated piece of research conducted by George Brown and Tirril Harris mainly in the London borough of Camberwell in the early 1970s.[8] In elaborating a causal model for the development of depression from their findings, Brown and Harris first stress the importance of how "provoking agents" precipitate a depressive episode, such as major life events and continuing difficulties. However, they found that these life events and difficulties were much more frequent and severe among working-class women than middle-class women; problems concerning housing, finance, husband, and children were particularly important. This imbalance in the experience of problems partly accounted for the large social-class difference in the incidence of depression, but most of this class difference was explained by the greater likelihood of a working-class woman having one or more of the four main "vulnerability factors," which determined whether or not a provoking agent would lead to depression. These vulnerability factors were having three or more children under fourteen at home, being unemployed, not having a trusting and confiding relationship, especially with a husband or boyfriend, and having lost her mother before the age of eleven. The factor of having young children at home was especially cogent, and working-class women in this position were four times more likely to suffer from a definite psychiatric disorder than similarly placed middle-class women.

Clearly, such factors as housing, employment, and facilities for the care of young children are outside the ability of a psychotherapist to alter, but it might be claimed that psychotherapy provides the trusting and confiding relationship that has shown to protect women from becoming depressed. But this ignores the obvious point that offering such a relationship to an already depressed woman is like shutting the stable door after this proverbial horse has departed. It could also be argued that the fact that many depressed women do not have an intimate friend with whom to discuss their problems is a comment on the dislocated and estranged quality of urban living. This argument would be supported by the finding, in a parallel study conducted in a rural community in the Outer Hebrides, that no such special vulnerability on the part of working-class women was observed; indeed, in the rural community there was no class difference in the incidence of depression of any kind. It is true that discussion of their feelings about the loss of their mothers may have helped those depressed women with whom this had occurred, but this is greatly outweighed in importance by the socioeconomic factors.

So far we have considered the findings of Brown and Harris only in respect to the risk of developing depression in the year of study. When chronic depression is considered, the lot of working-class women appears even worse. All forms of marked long-term environmental difficulties were more common among working-class women, and these were closely associated with physical health problems. Some of the difficulties, particularly concerning housing, had clearly served to perpetuate psychiatric conditions.

Overall, the survey by Brown and Harris found that no less than one third of the subjects interviewed showed evidence of a definite or borderline psychiatric condition. This is surely an indictment of the role women are required to play in industrial societies. Incidentally, these findings cast doubt on the conventional psychiatric distinction between "reactive" and "endogenous" depressions, since severe life events and major difficulties were associated with the onset of all types of depression, and specific clinical syndromes showing the presence or absence of provoking agents did not emerge from the analysis.

One reaction to the Brown and Harris findings might be to say that psychotherapists are well aware of the social and economic origins of many of the problems they deal with, but are nevertheless duty bound to try to provide relief for psychological distress. Let us see how far psychotherapists are in fact aware of this, by consulting the most authoritative source possible, The Handbook of Psychotherapy and Behavior Change and, in particular, the article by Raymond P. Lorion entitled "Research on Psychotherapy and Behavior Change with the Disadvantaged: Past, Present, and Future Directions."[9] Although this is a thoroughly researched, informative, and obviously well intentioned piece of work, it does contain some fundamental flaws in its discussion of the possibilities of psychotherapy for the disadvantaged.

Lorion tells us early in his article that many epidemiological studies have shown an inverse relationship between the distribution of psychological disorders and socioeconomic status. We have known this since the classic studies of A. B. Hollingshead and F. C. Redlich[10] with psychiatric patients and (L. Srole and others[11]) with a general population sample. Moreover, it is also well established that lower-class individuals are less likely to be accepted into treatment; less likely, if they are accepted, to be offered psychotherapy as opposed to physical treatments; and less likely even if offered psychotherapy to be treated by experienced therapists, who seem to prefer patients of their own class.

All this suggests that the most important issues to be considered in a discussion of psychotherapy for the disadvantaged are political, in the wider sense of the term. Psychotherapy may have some part to play in alleviating the psychological distress of the poor, but its contribution is limited. However, these obvious conclusions are nowhere to be found in Lorion's review. Instead we are told that "the business of mental health is to facilitate individual adaptation and adjustment to sources of psychological conflict."[12] If these sources are part of the condition of being, in Lorion's own words, "poor, depressed, incompetent, and powerless," then this presumably is the object of adjustment and adaption of psychotherapy.

What is interesting about Lorion's discussion is that he obviously has compassion for and some understanding of the lot of the poor and even a sense of indignation that they have been ignored by psychotherapists in the past. But in a strangely schizoid way, he makes no attempt to relate the objective conditions he mentions to a consideration of the role and limitations of psychotherapy.

Moreover, there is a further obfuscation in Lorion's use of the rhetoric of mental health, and this is where the analogy with the political context of physical disease breaks down. Although the origins of tuberculosis, for example, lie in damp and insanitary housing conditions, once one has contracted tuberculosis, one is in need of treatment and cure; the main relevance of the housing conditions is in prevention. If by using the term "mental illness" the impression is given that the problems that require psychotherapy are similar in kind, then a similar justification might be offered for psychotherapy with the socially disadvantaged. But this is seriously misleading, for often it is not merely the origins of problems experienced by the disadvantaged that are socioeconomic but the very nature of these problems. In many cases, they are not psychological problems as such, but social and economic problems. This is obscured in the rhetoric of mental health and illness.

I would not wish to press this argument too far by denying that psychotherapy has any relevance to the problems of the poor. Many psychotherapists realize the true nature of their clients' presenting problems but feel impotent to do anything about them; meanwhile, they attempt to make life more tolerable for the unhappy individual. I shall have more to say about this later, when I consider the personal dilemmas confronting the politically aware psychotherapist. Suffice it to say here that, although they cannot change the social and economic forces that bear upon the individual client's life, I believe psychotherapists should acknowledge frankly the limitations of their skills and then constantly reassert in their writings and discussions with colleagues and students the fact of the social injustice that so often makes their labors necessary.

PSYCHOTHERAPY AS A MYSTIFYING AGENCY OF SOCIAL CONTROL

I have not meant to suggest that psychotherapists' attempt to disguise the socioeconomic nature of human problems is deliberate. But however unintentional it may be, the disguise is clearly of benefit to the established social order. As well as offering a spurious adjustment to the discontented and potentially rebellious, psychotherapy can be seen as serving to stifle at the source a critical analysis of an existing social organization. It thereby helps to perpetuate the status quo and retard the possibility of fundamental social change.

This is roughly what is meant by claiming that psychotherapy acts as a mystifying agency of social control. Of course, all societies contain methods of controlling their constituent members, but the point about psychotherapy, and other "helping" professions like psychiatry and social work, is that they undertake mystifiying social control. This means more than merely "disguised" and "distorted," terms that have been used so far and it is more than merely a matter of providing misleading answers to critical questions. Mystifying social control presents social reality in such a way that the critical questions never arise or, if they do arise; are regarded as meaningless and inadmissible. The last section of this chapter emphasizes the results of poverty and other aspects of social injustice; this section goes beyond them. The concerns of the thinkers to be discussed here are equated with the destructive tendencies inherent in affluent mass society.

There are several levels at which psychotherapy can be viewed as a mystifying agency of social control, and I will begin with the most trivial level. The idea here is simply that the goals toward which psychotherapy is directed, and therefore the criteria under which it judges whether or not it has been successful, are taken from prevailing, dominant norms and values. However objective and "scientific" the psychotherapist attempts to be, it would be remarkable if his or her own normative standards, reflecting a high status as a representative of respectable middle-class morality, did not penetrate the negotiation of therapeutic goals. Normal, well adjusted family life or productive working relationships permeate the psychotherapeutic situation and exert a profoundly conservative influence.

This is now a familiar criticism of psychotherapy, and I will no longer labor the obvious except to say that, although trivial, it is no less worthy of our serious consideration.[13] Neither should it be thought that encounter groups and other forms of "liberating" and "self-actualizing" therapies evade the force of this simple criticism. Indeed, in its obsession with self-growth and private experience, the encounter group movement is diametrically opposed to seeking collective solutions to the alienation of modern life. One can do no better here than quote Sigmund

Koch's savage indictment of the group movement.

> The group movement is the most extreme excursion so far of man's talent for reducing, distorting, evading and vulgarizing his own reality. It is also the most poignant exercise of that talent, for it seeks and promises to do the very reverse. It is adept at the image-making manoeuvre of evading human reality in the very process of seeking to discover and enhance it. It seeks to court spontaneity and authenticity by artifice; to combat instrumentalism instrumentally; to provide access to experience by reducing it to a packaged commodity; to engineer autonomy by group pressure; to liberate individuality by group shaping. Within the lexicon of its concepts and methods, openness becomes transparency; love, caring and sharing become a barter of "reinforcements" or perhaps mutual ego-titillation; aesthetic receptivity or immediacy becomes "sensory awareness." It can provide only a grotesque simulacrum of every noble quality it courts. It provides, in effect, a convenient psychic whorehouse for the purchase of a gamut of well advertised existential 'goodies': authenticity, freedom, wholeness, flexibility, community, love, joy. One enters for such liberating consummations but inevitably settles for psychic striptease".[14]

The accusation that psychotherapy acts as an agency of social control can be interpreted, not only on the level of the practical consequences of individual or group treatment, but also on the level of the theories of human nature upon which the therapeutic method is based. Personality theories, besides supporting their associated therapies, have an independent life as contributors to the way in which human existence is understood, and especially, the way the individual is seen in relation to the surrounding society. Easily the most outstanding example of this is psychoanalytic theory, which, it has been argued,[15] has had a far greater effect on the world through the widespread dissemination of Sigmund Freud's ideas among intellectuals and artists than through the elitist practice of psychoanalysis. On this level, many radicals have deplored the reactionary trends in psychoanalytic theory, but against this, there is a long tradition in European thought devoted to the attempted marriage of Freudian and Marxist theory. No full account of the politics of psychotherapy can afford to ignore this tradition, but here I am able to provide no more than a suggestive outline of this immensely deep and complex subject.[16]

During the 1920s there were several attempts by leftist Freudians to integrate psychoanalysis and Marxism, probably the most notable being the work of Wilhelm Reich.[17] However, the most concerted and influential attempt to do so was made by the so-called Frankfurt School, associated with the names of Theodore Adorno, Max Horkheimer, and Hebert Marcuse. The "critical theory" of this school of thinkers has been described in 1973 by M. Jay[18] and utilized in 1975 by Russell Jacoby in his brilliant polemic, <u>Social Amnesia</u>.[19]

The need for an integration of Freud and Karl Marx arose from the failure of the revolutionary movement in Central Europe following the First World War and the continued existence of capitalist society, despite the fact that the "objective" conditions for its collapse apparently existed. This led to a dissatisfaction with a "vulgar" mechanical and purely economic Marxism and the need to add to an understanding of the objective conditions, the <u>subjective</u> conditions of social revolution. This led, in turn, to a rediscovery of the early philosophical Marx and to the Hegelian roots of Marxism, to the revival of a dialectical understanding of man in society, and to an interest in psychoanalysis as providing a theory of repression in class society and an account of the means by which the capitalist mode of production renews itself. Later Freudian theory was also employed, in an attempt to explain the horror of Fascism.

According to Jacoby, the revolutionary implications of Freud's own work have been repressed in later versions of psychoanalysis. He suggests that Freud's unremitting devotion to the truth overcame his personal, conservative predilections to reveal the essential contradiction between the individual and the demands of a repressive civilization. For Jacoby and the Frankfurt School, it is the ability of Freudian thought to pass beyond the surface of human experience and expose what was previously taboo--sexuality, the unconscious, the libido--that gives it its critical cutting edge.

Although Jacoby does not stress this point, it

was principally when psychoanalytic theory became "anglicized" from European into British and American hands that the repression of its subversive content occurred. This was achieved most notably by the elimination of Freud's "biologism" and the substitution of an emphasis on self and social adjustment by the neo-Freudians,[20] following the example of Mortimor Adler. For Jacoby, the so-called post-Freudians,[21] provided an even more flagrant illustration of a conformist psychology, located firmly in the tradition of a subjectivist, liberal ideology and designed to obscure the violence and destructiveness of late capitalism.

The point of departure for the Frankfurt School is clearly the idea that the repression that results in the discontents of civilization is not the inevitable consequence of <u>any</u> form of social organization, but is a specific consequence of the particular form based on the capitalist mode of production. It is the "surplus-repression" required by societies founded on class exploitation that is the chief cause of the defense mechanisms preventing healthy ego functioning. Moreover, in addition to pure biological instincts, the ego has also to deal with the demand of "second nature"--the accumulated and sedimented history of oppression. The Frankfurt School is especially concerned with the way in which the mechanisms of repression are contained in the mass culture of our times.[22]

What is the relevance of all this to the practice of psychotherapy? The most serious objection of the Frankfurt School to the neo-Freudians is that in attempting to strengthen the therapeutic practice of psychoanalysis, they had succeeded in weakening its theory. Innovations and revisions seen as necessary on pragmatic, therapeutic grounds are not objectionable in themselves, but they are objectionable if they have the effect of blunting psychoanalysis as a critique of society and turning it into little more than an instrument of individual adjustment.

Freud was acutely aware of the danger that his theory would be transformed into a mere system of psychotherapy. In advocating the contribution of lay analysts, he wrote that "the psychiatrist who takes up psychoanalysis is interested in the therapeutic needs chiefly. This aim is not to be disparaged, but it is not the main or even the essential aim of psychoanalysis. The chief aim of psychoanalysis is to contribute to the science of psychology and to the world of literature and life in general."[23] He also saw that the stripping of theory from psychoanalysis would be a peculiarly North American phenomenon. Extending the argument from psychoanalysis to methods of psychotherapy in general, these methods can always be judged by the degree to which they provide a coherent critical analysis of the socioeconomic conditions implicated in neurotic manifestations rather than merely to gloss over such matters.

Andrew Collier a more recent theorist and therapist, within the broadly defined psychoanalytic tradition, who could hardly be accused of merely summarizing the political content of Laing's views, runs into difficulties. However, Laing, as pointed out in his excellent study[24] adopted different positions at different stages of his career.[25] To quote from Jacoby; "though [his] thought genuinely resounds with political radicalism, revolutionary elan and theoretical coherence; yet it finally dribbles into blind therapy and positivism, pop existentialism and mysticism."[26] To do justice to Laing, it is necessary to emphasize his most coherent period during the early 1960s, in which he produced The Self and Others,[27] Sanity, Madness and the Family (in collaboration with Aaron Esterton),[28] and Reason and Violence (in collaboration with David Cooper).[29]

In one sense Laing's work is continuous with Freud's and avoids one of the important revisions of the neo-and post-Freudians. This is the position that there is a continuity between health and sickness and, hence, essential unity of psychic phenomena. This immediately makes it possible for Laing to describe the "pathology of normalcy," or the way in which adaptation to capitalist society entails, by definition, the adaptation of a false self to false realities. Later in his work, of course, this principle is pushed even further, to produce an exact reversal of conventional thought in which the mad are sane and the sane, mad. The psychotic breakdown is seen as akin to the experiential voyage of the mystic--as a departure from the alienation of normal life in order to discover the real self in a process of "existential rebirth." It is here, of course, that most serious radicals part company with Laing, regarding his advocacy of transcendental experience as merely futile escapism.

A further political strand in Laing's thought is concerned with his insistence on understanding madness as existing in systems, such as family units, rather than in individuals. This is illustrated by the case studies discussed in Sanity and Madness in the Family.[30] The trouble with this perspective is that it does not go far enough, since the family is presumably part of a larger system of more remote social relationships, until the level of the total society is reached. Laing was aware of this larger context and discussed it at length in several places.[31] However, family therapy that is based on the systems theory perspective fails to acknowledge the limitations revealed by these insights.

These criticisms of Laing should not be taken as denigrating his brilliant account of the phenomenology of the schizoid experience[32] and his important contribution to the methodology of psychiatric research. Unfortunately, however, the best that can be said for the political content of his ideas is that they exerted some influence on the "micropolitics" of student rebellions and hippy experiments during the 1960s. But we are now in a very different economic situation and the relevance of Laing's work to an understanding of the political context of psychotherapy can almost be dismissed as of only historical interest.

PSYCHOTHERAPY AS A MEANS OF FOSTERING DEPENDENCE ON BUREAUCRATIC INSTITUTIONS

At the beginning of this chapter I suggested that a common element running through various meanings of the term "politics" was that they all involved the concept of power, or "the means by which some people or groups acquire and maintain a greater control over the situation than others."[33] A recent discussion of the therapeutic relationship by I. Barofsky[34] begins with the assumption that all therapy is political in this sense because "at the core of the phenomenology of all patients is a sense of loss: a sense of losing personal control over oneself in order to become part of a system that is to restore health, but by unfamiliar methods. This loss of power seems to be the key event that justifies looking at the health care process as a political process".[35] Although Barofsky's concern is the wider area of relationships between doctors and patients, his remarks are especially relevant to psychotherapy. For example, Jerome D. Frank observed that the major source of the distress of persons who seek psychotherapeutic help is "a sense of failure or of powerlessness to affect oneself and one's environment".[36] However, the purpose of Barofsky's discussion is to establish how the therapeutic relationship can be structured so as to enable patients to liberate themselves from the passive-dependent roles in which they are normally cast and, thereafter, begin to develop forms of self-care.

This last position has been taken to its logical limits by Ivan Illich and his followers, and I will devote the rest of this section to their work. It should be noted at the outset, however, that this sort of criticism of psychotherapy comes from a very different political stance than encountered in the previous section. Here it is assumed that industrial societies have passed beyond the capitalist stage of development and have entered a new stage in which it is the technological process that determines the nature of social organization; and the managers of capital, the technocrats and bureaucrats rather than the owners, have control. Moreover, in this form of technological industrial economy, it is no longer possible to distinguish what used to be called capitalist from what used to be called socialist societies.[37]

THE DISABLING EFFECTS OF PROFESSIONAL SERVICE

In a book edited by Illich and others entitled Disabling Professions,[38] there is an article by John McKnight called "Professionalized Service and Disabling Help."[39] McKnight begins by stating that the business of modern society is service and that it is the needs and political interests of the professional service providers that have become paramount. Professionalized assumptions of need have three disabling effects.

First, the needs of citizens, which might be satisfied in any number of ways, are transformed by professionals into deficiencies with which only they can deal.

Second, mainly because the services available are usually limited to individual interaction, the deficiency is located inside the client rather than in the socioeconomic context. This is by now a familiar point, but, this time it implies that the available solution defines the problem, rather than the other way around. At this point McKnight praises the civil rights and women's liberation movements, which struggle to overcome the communications of personal deficiency from professional service ideology.

Third, the highly organized and intricate nature of service systems results in the specialized breakdown of the client's needs into a collection of problems. Thus the client's marriage problems may be dealt with by a marriage counselor, vocational problems by an occupational psychologist, drinking problems by an "alcohologist," and so on. The main effect of this compartmentalization of a person's problems is that it removes the potential for individual action.

In other words, service systems communicate the following three propositions to the client:

1. You are deficient.
2. You are the problem.
3. You have a collection of problems.

In terms of the interests of service systems and their needs, the propositions become as follows:

1. We need deficiency.
2. The economic unit we need is individuals.
3. The productive economic unit we need is an individual with multiple deficiencies.[40]

Professionalized definitions of needs produce a complementary set of remedial assumptions, with further disabling effects, as follows:

The Professional says to the citizen;

1. We are the solution to your problem.
2. We know what problem you have.
3. You can't understand the problem or the solution.
4. Only we can decide whether the solution has dealt with your problem.

In terms of the needs of professionalized service systems, these propositions become:

1. We <u>need</u> to solve your problems.
2. We <u>need</u> to tell you what they are.
3. We <u>need</u> to deal with them in our terms.
4. We <u>need</u> to have you respect our satisfaction with our own work.

First, mirroring the assumption that the problem lies within the client is the further assumption that only the professional can provide the answer, not the client or the client's peers or social environment. Also denied is the possibility that there is no answer. McKnight also refers to attempts by service providers to deal with the anxiety stemming from the need to deny the unilateral nature of relationships by calling them "community-oriented" or "client-oriented." He would presumably include client-centered psychotherapy in this.

The second corollary of professionalized definitions of needs arises from the necessity to define the need in terms of the available remedy. To ensure that the professional's highly specialized tools and techniques are fully employed, the client must understand that only the professional can understand what is deficient in him or her. Thus the professional arrogates the right to define what questions are appropriate, so that only the professional can provide the appropriate answers.

Third, as a consequence of this right, the problem and its solution are coded into a language that is incomprehensible to the client. In addition to being told that he or she is incapable of deciding whether or not there is a problem, it is also demonstrated that the client would not understand the problem or its solution anyway.

Fourthly, following from all these professional powers is the right of the servicers to unilaterally define whether the results of their service are satisfactory. Once more, the four communications of the professional to the citizen are matched by four corresponding communications of needs of service systems.

McKnight's critique of professional service, and indeed the entire attack on the bureaucratic institutions of modern industrial society, has many attractions. It gives voice to many of the diffuse and sometimes incoherent objections to the encroachment of the "caring" professions on personal liberties in Western Europe and North America over the last 20 years or so.[42] At the same time, it gives encouragement to the many kinds of self-help and mutual aid on the part of various oppressed and disadvantaged groups. These are aimed, quite properly, at the development of more power and control over their own destinies. It is possible, however, that McKnight's critique has greater relevance to the formal institutions of psychiatry and social work, within which varieties of psychotherapy admittedly play an important part, than to the practice of psychotherapy as such. It could be argued, in other words, that there is nothing intrinsically disabling about psychotherapy.

At one extreme, traditional psychoanalysis might

be regarded as a candidate for the most disabling form of psychotherapy, since as Andrew Treacher puts it, "it combines all the passively inducing characteristics of the traditional doctor-patient relationship with a remarkably pessimistic and activistic form of psychological determinism."[43] It should certainly not be imagined that, simply because much psychoanalysis has taken place on a fee-paying basis, it is therefore egalitarian and power sharing; nevertheless, it would be absurd to conclude that all forms of psychotherapeutic expertise are necessarily oppressive, especially since many of them appear to take the issue of the distribution of power in the therapeutic relationship as their point of departure from psychoanalysis.[44] Indeed, it is now nearly 40 years since the experiments of Maxwell Jones in Britain were specifically aimed at democratizing the interaction between treater and treated, although it is perhaps worthy of note that the therapeutic community movement within psychiatry is in sad decline.[45]

These examples show, I think, that the Illich position tends to produce a caricature of the therapeutic relationship rather than reveal anything essential. This caricature may point to very real dangers of the "therapeutic state," but it also contains some dangers of its own. McKnight's ideas may make more sense in the North American context in which they were conceived but in a country like Britain where a national health-care system was set up in defiance of fierce right-wing opposition, and where even now there are powerful forces directed at returning the provision of care to the marketplace, it seems perverse to suggest that professional services should be replaced by self-help. And it is highly significant that in North America it is the current leaders and architects of health policy who appear to have shown the most interest in the "therapeutic nihilism"[46] of the Illich school of thought. An example of this influence is the book _Healthy, Wealthy, and Wise_, edited by the president of the Rockefeller Foundation, John Knowles,[47] the chief message of which is that it is individual bad habits that are responsible for ill health. Thus the Illich and McKnight recommendations fall conveniently into the hands of the anticollectivist power establishment, which is searching desperately for ways to reduce spending on both physical and psychological therapies.

DILEMMAS CONFRONTING THE POLITICALLY ASTUTE PSYCHOTHERAPIST

During this rapid journey through the various intellectual positions that have made political criticisms of psychotherapy, perhaps one argument is shared by them all. This is that the practice of individual psychotherapy and the theories on which it is based tend to locate problems "inside" individuals rather than in the social systems in which the individual participates. Having arrived at this insight, however, what can the therapist do about it?

The immediate solution is obvious and is the one adopted by Treacher in his discussion of politics and psychotherapy.[48] It is to renounce the "clinical paradigm" from which individual therapy is derived and base intervention instead upon a systems theory approach that attempts to change the behavior, not of individuals, but of social systems. This approach does not include therapy with artificially assembled groups of strangers, since that merely recapitulates the clinical paradigm at a more sophisticated level. The social system most immediately relevant to the problems seen by psychotherapists is, of course, the family. It is my impression that among the many varieties of psychotherapy it is family therapy, or at least the version of it is imbued with a systems theory perspective, that has proved most attractive to politically aware psychotherapists. Not only does this approach come closer to an adequate set of assumptions about the causes of human problems, but it also avoids the iatrogenic labeling and processing of the arbitrarily selected individual and eschews the passivity-inducing imbalance of power inherent in the face-to-face situation.

A good example of such an approach is the work of the psychiatrist R. D. Scott at Napsbury, England, which is described by E. Bott.[49] Unlike Laing, whose views initially appeared similar, Bott has not turned his back on the National Health Service. However, the radical nature of his practice within the state system has led to his isolation among psychiatrists and the refusal of the <u>British Journal of Medical Psychology</u> until 1976 to publish any of his work.

It may be unnecessary to add here that the systems theory and crisis intervention approach by no means succeed in solving all the dilemmas faced by the politicized psychotherapist. The new set of conflicts that confronts therapists who have abandoned working with individuals has been well described by Philip Kingston:

> Knowledge about social influences on behavior places family therapists in two principal dilemmas. The first is that whilst such knowledge might indicate the necessity to change other systems, therapists have limited power to effect such change. Second, although collaboration with other systems may be necessary to bring about changes in the family, the cost of such collaboration may be the therapist's involvement in a process of control.[50]

The first dilemma Kingston refers to arises from the obvious fact that the family system, or any other "microsystem," is part of larger systems, which are in turn part of suprasystems, and so on up to the level of the total society. Although this had led some therapists to take on somewhat larger systems than the immediate family, an instance being C. Attneave's[51] work with tribal settings and urban network intervention, the sheer inter-relatedness of social problems has led others to abandon a political view of therapy. For example, from an ecological perspective, E. Auerswald[52] suggests that therapists should become "post-political" in order to avoid "the trap of politicization." Kingston[53] replies to this by arguing that any intervention in a system, including the family, is political, since it is aimed at changing or maintaining the balance of power or distribution of resources. In this sense, Auerswald's attempt to be "post-political" succeeds only in being "pre-political."

The limited extent to which the therapist can alter larger systems in order to effect changes at a smaller level, such as the level of families, raises Kingston's second dilemma. Quite simply, such attempts often smack of manipulation and seem to run counter to the objective of increasing people's control over their lives. There is clearly no simple and overriding solution to this kind of problem, but what seems important is that the assumption of control by the therapist, if occasionally it seems expedient, is always openly acknowledged and never mystifying.

Quite apart from dilemmas arising from direct contact with families and other systems, there exists another related set of dilemmas, involved with the institution that employs the therapist.

These dilemmas are best considered in relation to the following section which concludes this chapter.

POSSIBILITY OF A LIBERATING OR RADICAL PSYCHOTHERAPY

In this section I wish to examine the implications of the foregoing material for the practice of psychotherapy. I can provide no definitive answers to any of the problems raised. Where generalizations are deemed possible, I make most of them with hesitation. It is not so much a question of describing a path through the jungle of competing and conflicting points of view, as of merely warning against some of the dangers that may be encountered on the way.

Although the ideas reviewed in this chapter have been put forth in the context of the so-called developed nations of the world, some attention must be paid to the particular situations of developing nations. I will make these observations with diffidence because of my ignorance of the status and role of psychotherapy in the cultures of developing nations and because of my reluctance to be construed as giving anybody advice. Obviously, every culture must work out its own solutions to the problems raised by the politics of psychotherapy.

The term "liberating psychotherapy," usually prefixed by the adjective "genuinely," was frequently heard during the period of optimism about radical causes in the 1960s and early 1970s. The term is still relevant to our topic, because it offers the promise of somehow resolving all the dilemmas and conflicts arising from the interface of politics and psychotherapy. There can be no such thing as a liberating psychotherapy, "genuine" or otherwise.

The central charge that has been levelled against psychotherapy through all the various criticisms of it is that it "individualizes" problems the real origins of which are to be found in structures of the total society. It is impossible for psychotherapy ever to transcend these charges, which I take to be the implication of the word "liberating," since psychotherapy always takes place within the social structure. Liberation can only be achieved by changing the social structure itself.

As suggested in the last section, some people believe that this impasse can be broken simply by going beyond the individual in treatment and attempting to change social systems. The absurdity of this belief can be demonstrated by recalling the psychiatrist described approvingly by Laing whose "strategy was to reconvene the network out of which the mother has dropped in the past twenty years, eventually bringing together at one meeting upwards of thirty-five people, representing elements of no less then seven nuclear families. He did not treat the son or the mother individually, or as a dyad, but 'treated' the whole network".[54] But as Jacoby points out, even if such a number of people could be "treated," why stop there? "The implicit logic suggests the project of gathering all the members of society in one room, as if the antagonisms could be ironed out in the give and take of a group discussion".[55] Indeed, Laing does often write as though the project of changing society is of the same order as that involved in a difficult session of group (or family) therapy!

Another approach to a liberating psychotherapy by some radicals has been to devote their attention to raising the "political consciousness" of those with personal problems. An example of this approach was the Socialist Parents' Collective (SPK), which was set up in Heidelberg, West Germany, in 1970. This is hardly an example of concrete thinking, since it seems to assume that because the ultimate cause of a person's obsessional neurosis may exist in the guilt-inducing methods of childrearing found in capitalist societies, that person can be cured by a diligent reading of Marx and Engels. Apart from the absurdity of this, in West Germany any concerted attempt to put these ideas into practice, however harmless they may be, is unlikely to be tolerated by the state, as was shown by the fate of the SPK which was forcibly disbanded, with the psychiatrists involved receiving four-and-a-half-years prison sentences for "criminal association."

The promise of liberation is most closely associated with the radical chic of "alternative therapy," a term meant to include the hundred-and-one varieties of therapy that have proliferated outside the formal medical sector in the United States and, to a lesser extent, in Britain and other Western European countries and are available on a fee-paying basis on the open market. As Joel Kovel has remarked; "the half-life of therapies now comes to resemble that of schools of art or rock groups."[56] As such, they seem to have become an accepted part of modern mass culture and must compete with each other more and more vigorously. Tied in as they are with the vanities and self-indulgence of affluence, the relevance of these forms of therapy to the situation of developing countries appears to be nil.

My view of alternative therapy of this sort is closely akin to Koch's summary of the encounter group movement[57] previously quoted. The commercialization that has come to characterize these activities was potentially present from the beginning and leads not to liberation but to its very opposite: captivity by the most alienating forms of self-deception present in modern life. Moreover, as Peter Sedgewick puts it;

> Judged overall, however, the current expansion of private therapeutic practices, although often framed within a non-medical or even antimedical rationale, amounts to a trend very similar to that contained in privatized, fee-for-service medicine itself; it funnels money, skills and careers away from the severe and the chronic personal problems of the lower socioeconomic orders (who cannot foot the bill or speak the language of the more affluent private sector) and into the less chronic, less severe but financially rewarding and culturally voguish difficulties of the well-heeled. "Alternative therapy" is an alternative not so much to medicine, as to the social organization of health care according to need."[58]

As for the political content of alternative therapy, this may perhaps be summarized by the catch phrase on the cover of an issue, published in about 1970, of <u>The Radical Therapist</u>, the magazine that expressed the countercultural position on psychotherapy. It said; "Therapy means political change".[59] The shallowness of this view and of the confusion of the personal with the political has been demonstrated by subsequent history.

So *if* psychotherapy cannot be "genuinely liberating" or contribute to political change, what *are* the implications of the criticisms of psychotherapy reviewed earlier? Any positive answer to this question must be based on the assumption that the "reformism", that is, the attempt to bring about improvements, possibly limited and short term, while working within the system, is a worthwhile activity. Such attempts may be described as "radical" if they are consistent with, and indeed spring from, the same overall perspective as the desire for fundamental structural changes in society. The opposite view, that because these fundamental changes are not immediately forthcoming there is nothing to do but cultivate one's own garden, is of course a philosophy of despair.[60]

Although I have rejected talk of liberating psychotherapy as confused and misplaced, there are nevertheless themes present in such aspirations that are worthy of closer scrutiny. One is the move towards "demedicalization" of psychotherapy. As D. Ingleby[61] has remarked, psychoanalysis lost whatever radical potential it may have had when it became absorbed by the psychiatric wing of the medical profession. Interestingly, in France, where for historical reasons psychoanalysis has remained outside the gambit of medicine, it appears to have retained its radical message.[62] It is also interesting that Freud appeared to be quite aware of the dangers of absorbing his theory into medicine when he wrote; "We do not consider it at all desirable for psychoanalysis to be swallowed up by medicine and to find its last resting place in a textbook of psychiatry under the heading of 'Methods of Treatment'".[63]

I think this argument can be extended from psychoanalysis to psychotherapy in general, and some of the most interesting developments in psychotherapy since World War II can be seen as attempts to remove the elitist, authoritarian, or merely stultifying influence of the medical professional framework. It is difficult to say what could take its place. Clinical psychologists are hardly the most radical occupational group in Britain, and as Treacher[64] has remarked, they have either capitulated to medically created subservient roles or, in striking out on their own, have repeated the worst errors of the medical paradigm in an individualistic and mechanistic behavior therapy. Social work may hold more promise, but again, as far as Britain is concerned, is too encumbered with statutory responsibilities.

One advantage that both these groups have over medicine, however, is that they have a much shorter history as professions. I take it as axiomatic that the main characteristic of a profession is that it is organized to keep its specialized knowledge and power to itself and prevent them from falling into the hands of clients. In Britain there are strong forces seeking to "professionalize" clinical psychology and to limit the practice of psychotherapy to recognized groups with special training. One can sympathize with this to some extent because it is intended to remedy the invasion of people's lives by scientologists and the like. But this may be another example of an occupational group using the excuse of admitted abuse to increase its own power and control over an area. Radicals within psychology should fight against these tendencies, since it is still possible for them to put into practice George A. Miller's famous dream in his 1969 presidential address to the American Psychological Association of "giving psychology away."[65] With respect to developing countries, although I still wish to avoid the solecism of giving advice, one lesson from countries with a longer history of psychotherapy is that, while some medically qualified individuals may have much to offer as psychotherapists, if possible psychotherapy itself should be developed <u>outside</u> medical control.

Mention of the idea of giving psychology away, that is, of immediately sharing the discoveries of psychology and the power to influence lives that these discoveries bring about, raises the question, to whom should it be given away? For some years now there has been a movement to disseminate the skills of psychotherapy among lay persons, who can be relatively quickly and inexpensively trained to be effective therapists. Although there might be some discussion of how far paraprofessionals trained in psychotherapy become truly autonomous, there can be little doubt that this kind of development must be approved from the point of view adopted in this paper and would form part of any ideal organization of psychotherapeutic resources. However, it must be recognized that the principal reason for the spread of therapeutic skills is not that the spread is in the interest of the democratization of therapy; the principal justification relies purely on economic grounds, arising from an acknowledgment that future state funding will never be sufficient to train all the professionals who appear to be needed.

This economic justification coincides with the next logical step in the process of "giving psychology away," that is, giving it to those who themselves complain of psychological disorders. There is little doubt in my mind that the next big movement in psychotherapy, and in medicine generally, will be in the area of self-help. Indeed, there has already been a proliferation of self-help manuals for all kinds of psychological problems. But as I have pointed out, the movement toward self-help is attended by serious dangers. Sedgewick[66] has demonstrated that, paradoxically; it is the 1960s radical, liberatarian objections to professional activity, of which presumably the Illich school of thought is a later manifestation, that are now being used by conservative governments to cut back on resources for those in need.

At present this appears to be the central dilemma for a radical practice of psychotherapy. On the one hand there are real objections to the use of professional power and a laudable desire to increase people's control over their own destinies; on the other hand there is a reactionary movement towards a return to unfeeling and unjust laissez-faire in the provision of help for human problems. This is a difficult knot to untangle, and we are only just beginning serious consideration of it. One can point to a few general issues.

1. The need to distinguish between mutual self-help, in which the group is encouraged to apply its own solutions, and individual self-help, in which responsibility is merely returned to the isolated and helpless individuals;
2. The need to distinguish between the equivalent of "cure," for acute problems that may be amenable to self-help solutions, and "care," for chronic problems that may need continuing state provision; and
3. The levels and types of problem for which self-help is beneficial and not simply callous.

Since developing countries often face the consequences of exhaustion of public resources, self-help methods are expecially relevant to them.

The main conclusion to be drawn from the the political dilemmas facing the psychotherapist is that therapy is therapy and political activity is political activity and that the two should not be confused. As Sedgewick[67] insists, even though the remote causes of psychological disorders lie in the structure of society, there is nothing reactionary about providing help to the sufferer who requests that help. There is a distinction to be made between: (1) problems that are mainly economic, and (2) those with socioeconomic origins that have been overlaid by problems amenable to psychological and behavioral change. In the first case, therapy will be ineffective as well as inappropriate.[68] In the second case, it is sometimes difficult to know which should have priority, the economic or the psychological problems, but the latter may be relevant.[69] It must also be said that being politically aware does not exclude one from the ordinary duty of trying to ensure that people get the best treatment, in the sense of the most humane and potentially effective. Just trying to assure that people with problems, especially the poorer ones, actually receive psychotherapy, rather than having their brains and minds destroyed by electroshock and drugs, is itself a radical activity.

It would of course be asking too much to expect any general agreement about the political criticisms of psychotherapy, which have been very briefly and crudely summarized in this chapter, or any sort of consensus regarding the consequences for practice that flow from those criticisms. I shall be content, however, if I have succeeded only in raising these issues as legitimate subjects for discussion. I shall be satisfied, in other words, if I have merely put the question of the political context of psychotherapy on the agenda.

NOTES

1. R. D. Laing, The Politics of Experience, (New York: Pantheon, 1967).

2. This definition is given by H. H. Strupp, "Psychotherapy Research and Practice: An Overview," in S. L. Garfield and A. E. Bergin, (eds.), Handbook of Psychotherapy and Behavior Change, 2nd ed. (New York: Wiley, 1978), p. 3.

3. See for example T. McKeown, The Role of Medicine: Dream, Mirage or Nemesis, (Oxford, Blackwell, 1979).

4. This has now been published as P. Townsend and N. Davidson, Inequalities in Health, (Harmondsworth: Penguin, 1982).

5. See for example M. Muller, The Health of Nations: A North-South Investigation, (London, Faber and Faber, 1982).

6. The report was produced by the government's Central Policy Review Staff (colloquially known as the "think tank") in 1979 but has never been published. However, it may be obtained from Prof. Kettil Brunn, Studier in Svenska Alkohol Politik, Sociologiska Institutionen, Stockholm University, 5106 91 Stockholm. Insult was added to injury by

the subsequent publication of the almost completely ineffectual government discussion document, Drinking Sensibly, (London: HMSO, 1981).

7. For a discussion of this, see M. Tushen, "The political Ecology of Disease," Review of Radical Political Economics, (1977): 9, 45-60.

8. G. Brown and T. Harris, Social Origins of Depression: A Study of Psychiatric Disorder in Women, (London: Tavistock, 1978).

9. R. P. Lorion, "Research on Psychotherapy and Behavior Change with the Disadvantaged: Past, Present and Future Directions," in Garfield and A. E. Bergin, Handbook of Psychotherapy, pp. 903-38.

10. A. B. Hollingshead and F. C. Redlich, Social Class and Mental Illness, (New York: Wiley, 1958). This classic study has recently been repeated in the same area of New Haven and is described by F. C. Redlich and S.R. Kellert, "Trends in American Mental Health," American Journal of Psychiatry, 135: (1978): 22-28. The main finding in respect of the class bias in the incidence of psychiatric disorder was repeated, but there was a less clear distinction between the "physical" treatments given to working-class patients and the psychotherapy offered to the middle class.

11. L. Srole, T. S. Langer, S. T. Michael, M. K. Opler, and T. A. C. Rennie, Mental Health in the Metropolis: The Midtown Manhattan Study, (New York: McGraw-Hill, 1962).

12. Lorion, "Research on Psychotherapy," p. 904.

13. This criticism may be fleshed out somewhat by placing it in the context of social deviancy theory. See, for example, P. Conrad, "On the Medicalization of Deviance and Social Control," in D. Inglegy, ed. Critical Psychiatry: The Politics of Mental Health, (Harmondsworth: Penguin, 1981), pp. 102-19. For the argument that the deviancy analysis of psychiatry cannot be divorced from that of medicine in general, see I. K. Zola, "Medicine as an Institution of Social Control," Sociological Review, 20, (1972): 487-504.

14. S. Koch, "The Image of Man Implicit in Encounter Group Therapy," Journal of Humanistic Psychology, 11, (1971) 109.

15. See G. A. Miller, "Psychology as a Means of Promoting Human Welfare," American Psychologist, 24, (1969), 1063-75.

16. Possibly the key work is H. Marcuse, Eros and Civilization, (New York: Knopf, 1955).

17. See for example W. Reich, "Dialectical Materialism and Marxism," in Studies on the Left, 4 (1966), 6-7.

18. M. Jay, The Dialectical Imagination: A History of the Frankfurt School and the Institute of Social Research, (Boston: Beacon, 1973).

19. R. Jacoby, Social Amnesia: A Critique of Conformist Psychology from Adler to Laing, (Boston: Beacon, 1975).

20. The principal thinkers included under this rubric are Erich Fromm, Karen Horney, and Harry Stack Sullivan.

21. This usually refers to the work of Abraham H. Maslow, Gordon Allport, and Carl R. Rogers.

22. See Jay, Dialectical Imagination.

23. From S. Blanton, "Diary of My Analysis with Sigmund Freud", quoted in Jacoby, Social Amnesia, p. 123.

24. A. Collier, R. D. Laing: The Philosophy and Politics of Psychotherapy, (Hassocks, Sussex: Harvester, 1977).

25. This point is also made by P. Sedgewick, Psycho Politics, (London: Pluto, 1982).

26. Jacoby, Social Amnesia, p. 131.

27. R. D. Laing, The Self and Others, (London: Tavistock, 1961).

28. R. D. Laing and A. Esterton, Sanity and Madness in the Family, (London: Tavistock, 1964).

29. R. D. Laing and D. Cooper, Reason and Violence, (London: Tavistock, 1983).

30. Laing and Esterton, Sanity and Madness.

31. See for example R. D. Laing, "The Obvious," in D. Cooper, ed. The Dialectics of Liberation, (Harmondsworth: Penguin, 1968).

32. R. D. Laing, The Divided Self, (London: Tavistock, 1960).

33. G. Ponton and P. Gill, Introduction to Politics, (London, Martin Robertson, 1982), p. 35.

34. I. Barofsky, "Compliance, Adherence and the Therapeutic Alliance,: Social Science and Medicine, 12, (1978), 369-76.

35. Ibid., p. 369.

36. J. D. Frank, Persuasion and Healing, rev. ed. (Baltimore: John Hopkins University Press, 1973), p. xvi.

37. For a discussion of this, see V. Navarro, "The Industrialization of Fetishishm or the Fetishism of Industrialization: A Critique of Ival Illich," Social Science and Medicine, 9, (1975) 351-63.

38. I. Illich, Disabling Professions, (London: Marion Boyars, 1977).

39. J. McKnight, "Professionalized Service and Disabling Help," in Illich et al., Disabling Professions, pp. 69-91.

40. Ibid.

41. Ibid.

42. For an interesting discussion of the paradoxical effects of this libertarian tendency, see Sedgewick, Psycho Politics, pp. 187-256.

43. A. Treacher, "The politics of psychotherapy", New Forum, (Journal of the Psychology and Psychotherapy Association), 1977, no. 5. p. 63.

44. Included here would be George Kelly's personal construct psychotherapy, Rogers's client-centered therapy, and many later developments, culminating in the almost complete democratization found in Harvey Jackins's co-counseling method.

45. See D. H. Clark, Administrative Therapy: The Role of the Doctor in the Therapeutic Community,

(London: Tavistock, 1964).

46. This term is used in Navarro, "Industrialization of Fetishism."

47. Cited in L. G. Miller, review of J. Knowles, Healthy, Wealthy, and Wise, Social Science and Medicine, 12: 429-33.

48. Treacher, A. "The politics of psychotherapy", New Forum, (Journal of the Psychology and Psychotherapy Association), 1977, no. 5., p. 63.

49. E. Bott, "Hospital and Society," British Journal of Medical Psychology, 49, (1976), 97-140.

50. P. Kingston, "The Social Context of Family Therapy," in S. Waldrond-Skinner, ed., Family and Marital Psychotherapy, (London: Routledge and Kegan Paul, 1979).

51. C. Attneave, "Therapy in Tribal Settings and Urban Network Intervention," Family Process, 8, (1969), 192-210.

52. E. Auerswald, "Families, Change and the Ecological Perspecive," Family Process, 10, (1971), 263-80.

53. Kingston, "Social Context."

54. R. D. Laing, The Politics of the Family, (London: Tavistock, 1971), p. 49.

55. Jacoby, Social Amnesia, p. 138.

56. J. Kovel, "Therapy in Late Capitalism," Telos, 30, (1976) 73-92.

57. Koch, "Image of Man."

58. Sedgewick, Psycho Politics, p. 190.

59. Quoted in R. Kunnes, "How to Be a Radical Therapist,: in J. Agel, ed. Radical Therapist, (New York: Ballantine, 1971).

60. See the eloquent argument along these lines made in Sedgewick, Psycho Politics, pp. 243-45.

61. Ingleby, Critical Psychiatry, p. 61.

62. See for example S. Turkle, "French Anti-Psychiatry,: in Ingleby, Critical Psychiatry, pp. 150-83.

63. S. Freud, The Question of Lay Analysis, (New York, Basic Books, 1959).

64. Treacher, A. "The politics of psychotherapy", New Forum, (Journal of the Psychology and Psychotherapy Association), 1977, no. 5. p. 63.

65. G. A. Miller, 1969, address to the American Psychological Assn.

66. Sedgewick, Psycho Politics, pp. 187-256.

67. Sedgewick, Psycho Politics, p. 244.

68. Evidence for this statement is provided by E. Mullen and J. Dumpson, "Evaluation of social intervention," quoted in Kingston, "The Social Context of Family Therapy, " p. 53.

69. See the discussion of the work of Salvatore Minuchin and his colleagues in Philadelphia, who focus primarily on the family system itself, in Kingston, "The Social Context of Family Therapy," p. 55.

2

Traditional Therapies and Modern Therapies: Differences and Similarities

Michel Legrand

Communication among psychotherapists is difficult, in that it deals with extraordinarily ample and complex themes without access to the range of knowledge that could help in elaborating them. My ambition will be to open a few insights, even if these happen to end in a deadlock.

To understand anything about psychotherapies, it is of the highest interest not only to proceed with precise empirical research utilizing rigorous methodologies, but also to call upon the broad thought resources offered by anthropology and the human sciences from whom I will quote: ethnology, political science, history, and sociology, to name a few.

THE UNIVERSAL FIELD OF PSYCHOTHERAPY

Let us begin with ethnology. It is important to consider the phenomena that concern us, here, or "psychic troubles," and the ways to cope with them, ways present in all human societies, including societies sometimes still called primitive by ethnologists.

Georges Devereaux (1970; 1980), the founder of ethnopsychiatry, showed very well how "psychic troubles" are universal, recognized by all human cultures, and at the same time socially and culturally determined in terms of their generating mechanisms, structures, and problem resolutions.

Moreover, our reflection about psychotherapies would benefit from the following quote from Giovanni Jervis (1978): "It is likely that, since organized societies have existed, society asked some persons to specialize in solving anguishes and 'mind illnesses' and that such an aid was provided following technical channels of more or less 'institutionalized relationships'." On this point, I would like to mention the interesting works developed by the French Africanist School, and in particular the plan of African psychiatry developed in the School of Dakara, Senegal.

The modern Occident, then, did not discover "therapies," if we understand this word in this broad sense. However, it can be asked whether our modern therapies, in particular our psychotherapies, are different from the therapies of traditional societies. This will be the crux of my investigation. First, I will try to distinguish some differences between traditional and modern therapies; second, some possible likenesses.

DIFFERENCES: HOLISM AND INDIVIDUALISM

Holism

The French anthropologist Louis Dumont proposed a distinction that may be useful. He first studied the Hindu caste system, on which he wrote a book entitled Homo Hierarchicus (1967), which led to an examination of modern societies and their ideologies in Homo Aequalis (1977). Dumont distinguished two forms of societies: holistic and individualistic. On the one hand, traditional societies organized by the system of values he calls holistic are characterized by the privilege of the social whole and by the individual whose existence is dependent on the position occupied in the hierarchical social order. By contrast, modern societies are organized through an "individualistic" system of values, characterized by the privilege of the individual within the social whole, the latter finding its justification in allowing for the happiness and realization of the individual. No more social transcendence, no more sacred order.

If Dumont's distinction between holism and individualism is relevant, and if therapies are always caught in sociocultural forms, then this distinction must be able to enlighten the field of differences in psychotherapies. From it we can formulate the following macrohypothesis: therapies in traditional societies are holistic therapies, and therapies in modern societies are individualistic. And it is right to consider traditional therapies as adapted to a social universe dominated by holistic values. This claim is substantiated in the analysis by M. Auge and A. Zempleni (1975-76), two ethnologists of the French Africanist school. How do some African societies explain "psychical troubles" (or, more exactly, "bad-looking conditions") that cause their members suffering? For those societies, "psychical troubles" are caused by a social disorder; something has been disturbed in the network of social relations. So therapy is a restoration of social norms and of the position that each must occupy in the social whole. Therapy is holistic.

The Individual

By contrast, are modern therapies "individualistic"? What is the "individual"? What has caused this historical emergence?

To give a definition of the individual, I will use a distinction between person and individual proposed by the Brazilian anthropologist Roberto Da Matta (1978). The person is the human being, defined by that human being's position in a network of social relations; the human being is a member of a group, that is, a sexual group, age group, family group, caste, or social class. We can call the person an "affiliated" human being, and we can say that traditional holistic therapies are fundamentally therapies of the person. The individual, on the other hand, is the human being without organic links to the social whole. The human being who has identity or value independent of this position is in a network of social relation; this is the human being we can call "disaffiliated." Societies of disaffiliated human beings do not make a distinction between psychical troubles and organic or somatic troubles, because they do not separate body from mind.

The historical emergence of the individual represents an extraordinary but at the same time ambiguous achievement. There is a duplicity in the individual, the clear side and the dark one, the noble and the barbarian. The noble side is democracy; the barbarian, modern totalitarianism. This duplicity reveals the ambiguity of the idea of equality for the individual human being as the naked human being, equal to any other, the human being who contains value and absolute dignity beyond all barriers of race, class, and sex. But the individual human being, equal with others, is also the interchangeable, depersonalized, anonymous human being. The Occident has invented both democracy and the most barbarous forms of totalitarianism and violence, such as concentration camps. Soon we will see the impact of this duplicity in the field of psychotherapy.

How can we explain the historical emergence of the individual? It is too broad a subject to be given a thorough treatment here. Several hypotheses have been proposed, among which are those of the French sociologist E. Durkheim, with which I am in disagreement. Curiously, perhaps Marxism gives us the most satisfactory hypothesis. In fact, I believe that democracy is a fundamental historical and political form to which Marx did not give enough attention. It is probably the capitalist mode of production and the capitalist institutions of the market and the wage earners (i.e., the purchase and selling of the work force) that produced the individual. One can rediscover Marx's embryonic formulations of the individual in the Communist Manifesto. According to him, capitalism destroys all the social linkages of allegiance; this revolutionary virtue sets up the universal human being, the individual, the personified proletarian. This proletarian is the naked worker, the uprooted human being, and becomes the object of the market, the object of transactions, and is able to speak in the name of all the human beings, regardless of social, sexual and racial identity.

Before I address our modern therapies, I would like to bring out a distiction borrowed from my friend Robert Franck, a Belgian philosopher, whose important works concern the social significance of psychology (1983-84). This distinction is: The individual human being is divided, at once object and subject. This division is observed, for example, in the institution of wage earning, which may be the matrix of the process of individualization. In fact, the wage earner is an object, an entity of forces, an entity of objectified capacities, the work force (Marx), sold and bought at the market. At the same time, the wage earner is an autonomous subject, free to work or not to work, because he is not a slave, in some degree he remains owner of his work force and able to recover it in certain circumstances. Otherwise, the wage earner is divided into two parts, one of which is that objectified part that is given up or forsaken to the employer for a wage, and the other is that part of the wage earner that escapes the process of work, which the individual keeps: that person's thought, aspirations, and will.

Does this not evoke for all of us--psychologists, psychiatrists, and psychotherapists--something familiar? Are not our sciences and our other disciplines everywhere stamped by this polarity of the individual as object, including in modern medicine, which probably represents the most radical enterprise of objectification of the human being and subject (self, ego, and so on)?

Therefore, the most simple thesis we can maintain in connection with modern devices of curing psychic troubles would be that these devices will fit exactly the general character of modern culture. They are involved with this new social principle of the individual under two forms: "object" and "subject."

To test this thesis, we should turn to history. In the French cultural context, we have excellent historical works on the birth of psychiatric institutions, in particular Michel Foucault's books (1961; 1973). The problem is being rethought for the notion of "individual" and its historical emergence, as described by Marcel Gauchet and Gladys Swain (1980).

Franck asks himself why psychology was introduced in the field of madness. But from the moment when madness can no longer speak about social order and a religious, sacred universe, what can madness speak about except the individual under his or her double bind? The individual-object, the objectified body, the dark face of barbarism are all expressed in the most cruel violence practiced on the mentally ill. If there is a struggle to undertake, a struggle to lead in our field, let us not miss the target. Let us not attack psychotherapies, but mental hospitals and psychiatric hospitals. And I have to acknowledge the remarkable movement of Italian alternative psychiatry, which made a frontal attack on mental hospitals and carried out substantial changes in psychiatric care (LeGrande, 1988). On the other hand, the "moral treatment," one of the first forms of psychotherapy to which the French alienist movement gave its name, has had fundamental significance in questioning madness and in its connection with subjectivity. In any case, it is what Swain attempted to demonstrate in her book <u>Le sujet de la folie</u> (1977). Swain points to Franz Mesmer's practice as another source of modern psychotherapies, a source of what we could call the psychoanalytic therapies. These became possible when objectified medicine was born. Since the human body was objectified, all the subjective, imaginary, and fantasized aspects of the individual were rejected as irrelevant, as if the subject--object and individual--appeared at the same time in a process of dissociation.

THE UNIVERSAL PRINCIPLES OF THE FUNCTIONING OF THERAPIES

So far I have discussed the historical variations of therapeutic forms in terms of the distinction proposed by Dumont between holistic and individualistic societies; now I would like to follow a second line of reasoning that may not be very well coordinated with the first. Having examined the differences between traditional and modern therapies, let us examine their similarities.

Are there common principles at the basis of all forms of therapy? This is the classical question to common factors. To approach it, a metatheory is required. But what is this metatheory? There is much discussion of a new systematic paradigm. One of my colleagues, Candido da Agra, has published a thesis (1986) in which he defends the hypothesis of an actual reorganization of knowledge, biological knowledge as well as psychological and sociological knowledge, around a systematic paradigm. I would like to submit an approach to the problem of common factors, contained in this systematic paradigm. It is the approach of Jean-Marie Lacrosse (1984), a Belgian sociologist with whom I am working.

Her approach articulates a theory of psychic troubles, of therapies and of their respective efficacy. Each psychic trouble is translated into a paradoxical expression. Here there is a generalization of the well known theory of the "double bind" ("double link" or "double constraint") initially formulated by Gregory Bateson and others (1956) to account for schizophrenia and afterwards popularized by the Palo Alto School. To transcend the paradoxical expression, we must pass through at a metalevel. This metalevel will be brought about by therapy. Each therapy will give sense to symptoms and foster the disappearance of the symptoms from a metalevel discourse. From this, there follows four principles of functioning for healing the disease:

1. The principle of homeopathy, of healing the same by the same;
2. The principle of unrecognition of arbitrariness;

3. The principle of homogeneity between the context and global cultural symbolism, on the one hand, and the symbolism in which therapy is expressed, on the other; and
4. The principle of lack of progress.

I would like to comment individually on each of these four principles, specifying first that these are new hypotheses and are still provisional formulations.

Homeopathy

Homeopathy is a provisional metaphor that should probably be abandoned. It means that the symptom must be replayed or reproduced in the therapy. In fact, the symptom must be reproduced in order to be reframed later on.

The Unrecognition of Arbitrariness

Unrecognition of arbitrariness is the principle that states every therapy proceeds one way or another from a frame of reference within a belief system from which the symptom can be reframed. This belief system is arbitrary in the sense that it is neither right nor wrong. "Arbitrary," however, does not mean "whatever belief"; it means that the therapy system had best be drawn from the cultural forms in which the client participates.

Cultural Homogeneity

You cannot exorcise a Parisian intellectual; neither can you participate in psychoanalysis with an African pygmy. The principle of cultural homogeneity is that therapies draw their character from pre-existing sociocultural forms.

Lack of Progress

If therapy follows the first three principles, then it cannot improve. The historical development of therapies--their emergence, erosion, and renewal--does not enter into technoscientific logic, that is, a logic of cumulative progress (Frank, 1961). The development of medical technologies illustrates this point.

From these formulated propositions, two hypotheses can be put forward. The first has been formulated by LaCrosse: In a modern society focusing on recognition, on demystification, the belief systems cannot last for a long time. New belief systems are proposed again and again.
The second, different but not incompatible with the first, is drawn from Freud: If psychotherapeutic dispositions are connected with the problems of people (and since they must in some way reproduce those dispositions), then when problems change, dispositions must also change. Yesterday I formulated the hypothesis that psychoanalysis reproduces elements of a middle-class familial scene during Freud's era. It was suitable to the revival of the Oedipus drama. It can be understood that from the moment problems change, and are no longer Oedipal due to a global social evolution, the therapeutic dispositions must also change.

Many other things could be said about this theory; however, this is just a beginning. It seems to me essentially an opening to discussions, because it is essentially questionable. Many of us will not be able to relate to it. It privileges the model of myth and exorcism. But are not some of our modern therapies fundamentally mythologic practices? Could not therapies like psychoanalysis, bioenergy, and primal scream be reinterpreted in this way?

In my effort to confront traditional and modern therapies in the light of some approaches drawn from the human and social sciences, I followed two paths: the path of differences and the path of similarities. If each therapy is functioning with myths and beliefs, then no doubt it is functioning with contemporary cultural beliefs, that is, religious mythologies for holistic societies and individual mythologies for individualistic societies.

REFERENCES

Auge, M., and A. Zempleni. 1975-76. "Déviance quotidienne et totalitarisme ordinaire; Mal de soi, mal de l'autre", Autrement, no. 4: 203-16.

Bateson, G., D. Jackson, J. Haley, and J. Weakland. 1956. "Towards a theory of schizophrenia", Behavioral Science, 1, no. 4: 251-63.

Da Agra, C. 1986. Science, maladie mentale et dispositifs de l'enfance, Du paradigme biologique au paradigme systémique, Lisbon; Instituto Nacional de Investigaçâo Cientifica.

Da Matta, R. 1978. Carnavais, malandros e herois. Rio de Janeiro: Zahar.

Devereaux G. 1970. Essais d'ethnopsychiatrie générale. Paris: Gallimard.

Devereaux G. 1980. Basic Problems of Ethnopsychiatry. Chicago: University of Chicago Press.

Dumont, L. 1967. Homo Hierarchicus. Paris: Gallimard.

Dumont, L. 1977. Homo Aequalis, Paris: Gallimard. In English; From Mandeville to Marx: The Genesis and Triumph of Economic Ideology. Chicago: University of Chicago Press.

Foucault, M. 1961. Histoire de la folie à l'Age Classique. Paris: Plon.

Foucault, M. 1973. Madness and Civilization: A History of Insanity in the Age of Reason. New York: Random House.

Franck, R. 1983-84. "La signification sociale de la psychologie", Perspectives, 1-4.

Frank, J. 1961. Persuasion and Healing. Baltimore: Johns Hopkins University Press.

Gauchet, M., and G. Swain. 1980. La pratique de l'esprit humain. Paris: Gallimard.

Jervis, G. 1978. "A que serve la terapia?" In Il buon Rieducatore. Milan: Feltrinelli.

LaCrosse, J. M. 1984. "Sens et négociation dans la psychothérapie." Unpublished manuscript.

Legrand, M. 1988. La psychiatrie alternative italienne: Entre mythe et réalité. Toulouse: Privat.

Swain, G. 1977. Le sujet de la folie. Toulouse: Privat.

3

The Social Significance of Psychotherapy

Paul L. Wachtel

The potential range of questions that could be addressed by a chapter on the social significance of psychotherapy is enormous, and I can cover only a portion here. My focus in this chapter is not on the practice of psychotherapy per se, nor on the question of the social impact of that practice in itself. In a developing country, numerous questions need to be addressed concerning the appropriate psychotherapy for the poor and uneducated who do not share the attitudes or the social and economic position of the patients for whom the major therapeutic systems were first devised. There are many in my own country, also, who do not have the privileges one might expect in an "advanced" country, and I intend to follow closely the work of those who have worked in the so called third world.

In my own chapter, however, I will be mainly concerned not with practice, but with the values and assumptions that seem to be implicit in most psychotherapeutic systems. I want to look at the assumptions, habits of thought, and conceptions of human nature that lie behind the dominant approaches to psychotherapy.

As many commentators have noted, the evolution of the Western world during the last few centuries has been marked by a decline in the dominion of religion. The influence of such secular institutions as science and medicine have correspondingly expanded to fill the vacuum. In more recent years, psychotherapy and the theories that underlie it have played an increasing role in people's efforts to find meaning in their lives and to reconcile their conflicting desires with their ideas of what is right and proper. In the United States, and increasingly in other parts of the world as well, psychotherapists have come to function almost as a secular priesthood. The ideas that we therapists offer about the human condition have an impact that goes well beyond the effect on our individual patients. They contribute to molding the way people in our society view themselves and the way they conceive of human possibilities, desirable aims, and the appropriateness of various kinds of conduct. It is for this reason that I believe it so important to understand better what are the values and assumptions embodied in the dominant psychotherapeutic systems.

Discussions of matters related to psychotherapy tend to be couched in language that has a scientific and objective tone. Whether it be about the forces and energies of the Freudians or the stimuli and responses of the behaviorists, the typical language of psychotherapeutic discourse tends to obscure the role of values and of fundamental philosophical predilections. If we are to understand more fully the impact of our theories and practices on society, we must seek the unspoken assumptions that lie behind this language of objectivity.

I wish to focus particularly on a cluster of ideas and assumptions that underlie much of our thinking about psychotherapy and mental health. To begin with, I want to call attention to our use of the word "growth" in psychological discourse, our tendency to speak of the growth of the personality or of people growing through psychotherapy.

If we look closely, the word "growth" as used to describe the psychological development of a human being appears to be a peculiar phrase, although we are all in the habit of using it. Consider the physical growth of a human being, or of any creature for that matter. Certainly growth is very important during a period of our lives. We all begin life very small, and for a substantial portion of our lives we keep getting bigger and bigger; that is, we grow. But for an even longer period we do not grow; we maintain the same size and the same form. The adult's body maintains a dynamic equilibrium in which new cells are constantly being produced, but in which these new cells do not add to the size of the body but simply replace other cells that have died. Indeed, despite its providing us with the root metaphor for equating growth with development, the body also provides us with a cautionary image regarding an overemphasis on growth as a goal: When it is exclusively growth that continues to characterize some aspect of our bodily functioning, rather than dynamic equilibrium, what we have is cancer, our most feared disease.

Could it be that our use of the growth metaphor in psychological discourse derives at least in part from the strong emphasis on the idea of growth in our economic system? In what follows I want to consider how the nature of the society in which modern psychotherapy developed may have influenced the nature of our therapeutic systems. Such a consideration of the shaping influence of the economic basis of society was, of course, central to the thinking of Karl Marx. But one can see a similar strand of analysis in the writings of Erik H. Erikson, especially in his analyses of the way various aspects of the child rearing practices, values, and dominant modes of personality of different American Indian tribes could be understood as closely related to the way they earned their daily bread (or salmon, or bison).

In pursuing the task of relating aspects of our thinking about psychotherapy to our economic system and its ideological underpinnings, I will focus initially on the psychoanalytic tradition; partly because I find it easiest to; this is the tradition in which I was first trained, and the habits of thought of which probably still form the deepest layer of my professional psyche. Also, it has almost certainly been the most influential viewpoint guiding social criticism--as well as the therapeutic point of view most frequently the object of such criticism. Notions derived from psychoanalysis can even be seen to underlie many of the trends in psychotherapy that arose in opposition to psychoanalysis. For example, most of the "humanistic" therapies, from the pioneering work of Carl R. Rogers to the vast proliferation of humanistic approaches in the 1960s and 1970s, are characterized by some of the same underlying assumptions and habits of thought that I will be addressing in my consideration of psychoanalysis. Even where my argument focuses most explicitly on psychoanalysis, it can be seen as relevant to these other therapies as well.

Although Sigmund Freud's work has justly been described as presenting considerable challenges to the status quo of this society, there are also important (and not always noticed) ways in which his thinking served to maintain the status quo more effectively. Many commentators have noted that Freud's thinking was strongly influenced by the dominant scientific models of his day, by the science of forces and energies, which was built largely around the structure of classical mechanics.

Less frequently explored has been the influence of the social and economic ideas that were current then. Perhaps this is because it is easier to gain some distance from the worldview of nineteenth century physics. Physics, while not flatly contradicting the physics of Freud's student years, certainly provides us with a rather different set of dominant metaphors.

To be sure, economic and social thought have also advanced over the years, but like all the social sciences, their progress has been slower. Some of the social ideas that dominated in the years when Freud's theories were taking shape are still influential today. Indeed, they so permeate our own milieu that it may be difficult even to recognize them as specific assumptions rather than just "what is." This makes it very hard to recognize their specific shaping influence on our psychological theories, because they have had a shaping influences on all of us as well.

I would like to focus particularly on the individualistic nature of Freud's conceptualizations about human behavior and on their relation to the fundamental premises in our newspapers. At a U.S. Presidential news conference, one appreciates the centrality in our society of an image of people as discrete entities who search for their own profit and gratification. Society, from this viewpoint, is a pale shadow located behind these individuals; it provides the arena for their individual efforts but has little role in determining what those efforts will be.

The fundamental assumptions underlying a market economy such as ours correspond to a significant premise of many of today's dominant therapeutic systems. The latter, in conformance with the former, assumes that the sources of human motivation and human choices are best understood as deriving from deep within ourselves, rather than as significantly shaped by social forces. Within the economic sphere these assumptions are derived from an essential premise (false, in my opinion) that the constantly multiplying wants that characterize people's lives in advanced industrial societies are not an artifact of the values and economic arrangements of our particular system (i.e., of advertising, the need to "create" jobs in order to prevent unemployment, etc.), but a simple expression of human nature.

This set of assumptions has yielded us a constellation of grave problems, both social and ecological. Over the decades, our material standard of living has increased, but our personal satisfaction with what we have has not shown a corresponding rise. Indeed, through the 1970s, when per capita income in the United States was rising rather steadily (after correcting for taxes and inflation), there was a widespread perception of economic decline; people who were feeling they could barely make ends meet in fact had considerably more than their parents had at the same age or than had been typical when John Kenneth Galbraith could describe us, to general assent, as an "affluent society" (Wachtel, 1983).

The assumptions by which we are living have led to increasing discontent, even as the economy grows, and to a corresponding increase in selfishness and social regression. They have led us as well to stress continuing expansion of our industrial output, in a futile effort to keep up with the desires our way of life generates. Such ceaseless striving after more has taken an enormous toll on our life sustaining environment. Three Mile Island, Love Canal, PCBs, acid rain, dioxin--all have become unwanted additions to our vocabulary. Yet trapped in this way of seeing things, we experience no alternative to the relentless striving after economic growth except severe deprivation.

One might hope that psychotherapists, whose work involves studying the illusions that contribute to needless misery and investigating the genuine sources of satisfaction in people's lives, would at least in a small way contribute to combating those aspects of our modern worldview that lead us away from real satisfaction and into a labyrinth of self-deceptions and false solutions. Yet, in significant ways, the theories that guide therapeutic systems actually tend to reinforce the modes of thought which are at the heart of our social and ecological dilemma.

To be sure, we should not over estimate our capacity, in our role as psychotherapists, to affect large social events. Those who hold economic and political power clearly shape our society far more than we do; but we are not completely without influence. As noted above, our theories have partially filled the vacuum left by the decline of traditional religious beliefs. Our ideas do have an impact; for better or worse they seep into the sea of general social assumptions and give it a particular coloration.

But far more than we usually realize, by its nature our influence serves to maintain rather than combat the social patterns in which we are trapped.

The proliferation of desires that characterizes our way of life gains legitimacy to the degree that we view our desires as spontaneous upwellings of human nature and minimize their also being a product of our social system. Theories that stress internal determinants of behavior lead us to play down the role of social influences, whether they be the attitudes, expectations, or manifest behavior and way of life of friends or neighbors or the impact of advertising, the job market, or the nature of housing and transportation. These influences play an enormous role in what we think we want for ourselves, but they find little place in most of the theories that guide the work of psychotherapists.

The individualistic biases inherent in most approaches to psychotherapy are evident in many ways. In stressing autonomy, for example, as a possible and desirable goal for human beings, our theories contribute to the illusion that our desires and attitudes can be in a class by themselves. Ours is a society that overemphasizes independence as a characteristic of the successful and well functioning individual. This not only leads us to be unsympathetic to those in need, but also contributes to our dominant tendency to prefer individual ownership to sharing. The stress on the unattached single-family house as the ideal, with the concomitant necessity (and desire) for each of us to have our own washer, dryer, and so on, is part of a larger set of attitudes that contributes to our ecological crisis, requiring more and more to be produced. Our stress on independence also provides unfertile ground for an understanding of the interdependence that lies at the heart of an ecological point of view.

Psychotherapists are, of course, not responsible for the entire configuration of attitudes in our society; and an interpretation of independence and autonomy that is fundamentally opposed to interdependence is at least in part a distortion of what is intended by most of the psychological theories that rely on those concepts. Nonetheless, the stress on autonomy and on looking inward for the sources of our behavior does little to counter the prevailing trend and is likely to contribute in some ways to strengthening it, even if there are complex technical interpretations of the concept that do not strictly conform.

The same may be said regarding the emphasis on differentiation and separation--individuation that is also at the heart of much current therapeutic thinking. Ours is a society in which, to a degree that once would have been unimaginable, people are expected to move away from their families of origin and usually even from the communities in which they were raised. There is a strong confluence between these tendencies and the tendency to outgrow our possessions and require new ones constantly (see Wachtel, 1983, for a fuller discussion of these connections). And clearly there is a strong link between the latter tendency and the present strain on our environment. There has been increasing recognition among critically oriented therapists of the predisposition toward blaming of parents inherent in the major therapeutic approaches and of the bias toward separation from family as a sign of mental health. Once again there are more complex and sophisticated versions of the point of view under discussion here, versions that attempt to incorporate both the need for separation and the need for connection and reconciliation. But if we look not at the fine point but at the overall vector, we can see again how the views we promulgate are consonant with the major trends of the society at large.

It could, of course, be argued that the connotations and potential implications of our theories must take a back seat to their validity: If our theories are correct, then it is shortsighted to censor them because some of what they suggest is socially inconvenient. We will ultimately achieve a sounder basis for social justice and harmony with nature if our efforts are based on a correct assessment of human nature than if we try to pretend we are something other than what we are.

In response, several lines of argument are relevant. To begin with, we may note the rather tentative state of our knowledge at this point. Although psychological theories are often presented, all of them remain highly speculative. Much more evidence is required before we can even begin to argue that any particular theoretical position must be regarded as "the harsh truth," like it or not.

Indeed, an increasingly influential group of critical observers (see, for example, Habermas, 1971) have argued that it is in principle impossible to attain a view of human nature that is independent of the blinders and particular interests that place limits on any theorist, simply because that theorist is a member of a particular society and class and lives in a particular historical era. According to this view, any psychological theory will reflect not just some objective reality, but also the particular vantage point of the observer. Appreciation of the way the theorist's psychological conceptions serve to bolster or challenge the dominant social order is thus seen not as some external judgment brought to bear on a theory arrived at simply with the truth in mind, but rather something intrinsic to understanding what the theory, or any theory, is really about.

We may also note, in a different vein, that in fact an alternative to the highly individualistic theories of Freud and the various "humanistic" approaches exists, and that the alternative is capable of accounting for the same set of observations within a framework that has social implications that are considerably different. I am referring to the theories generally described as "neo-Freudian," which were quite influential some decades ago but have declined in influence in recent years.[1] The theories of Karen Horney, Harry Stack Sullivan, and Erich Fromm, supplemented by those of Erikson (who is not usually grouped with the other three, but who shares a number of their important views) provide the basis for a view of human behavior and experience that is better able to challenge the prevailing attitudes and habits than does orthodox Freudianism or the currently influential object relations theories.[2]

There are features of some of these theories that I find problematic, but by building upon them one can construct a theory that takes full account of the value and uniqueness of the individual and the individual's subjective experience but that does so in a way that fully integrates the individual's responsiveness to the world. Such an orientation does not conceive of an internal world split off from the events of the person's daily life, but rather presents the world of subjective experience and the world of environmental events as in continuous reciprocal interaction. Our subjective experience and behavioral inclinations are shaped by what happens in our daily lives, but the environmental events to which we respond are themselves in large measure determined by our own behavior and the behavior it elicits in others.

This type of theory presents an opportunity to employ psychodynamic insights in the service of a critique of the individualistic thinking that characterizes both classical psychoanalysis and the neoclassical economics that presently delimits our society's view of what is possible or desirable. The blather about "freedom to choose" (Friedman and Friedman, 1980) that currently passes for respectable social thought is leading us rapidly toward ecological disaster. As the late British economist Fred Hirsch (1976) noted in his perceptive analysis of the fallacies regarding economic growth, our efforts to solve our social problems individualistically are comparable to the efforts of a man who is standing in a crowd to see better by standing on his toes. Thinking just of what he can do alone, such a course of action seems to make perfect sense. He will indeed see better on his toes than not. But of course he is not likely to be the only one to think of standing on his toes. Others, too, will attempt this individualistic solution, either in an effort to gain some improvement in their situation or, after not too long, defensively in response to the fact that people in front of them have done so. The net result of all this will be that very few will have a better view than before, but that everyone will be more tired from the effort of standing on tiptoe (and unable to stop doing so because of the positive disadvantage it would now entail in the face of everyone else's doing so).

Much of what we face today fits well with Hirsch's paradigm. In an atmosphere in which we are encouraged to "look out for number one," we all end up exhausted but ungratified. The varied, and generally unrecognized, ramifications of this social pattern are beautifully elaborated in Hirsch's book.[3] Particularly in an era in which the ecological consequences of our multiple individual choices are so enormous, it is urgent for us to find a way to achieve collective solutions to our problems that are not subject to the ironies of the individualistic course. Yet it is equally essential to avoid the converse danger of the loss of freedom that has characterized those countries whose regimes have elevated collectivism to a monolithic principle, in which individual experiences and desires are given short shrift. Here is precisely where a psychological perspective that is attentive to the subjective needs of the individual yet alert to the nature of our profound interdependency, can prove useful. Such a psychology would not be an alternative to political and social action but a guide and spur to such action and a guarantor of its humane direction. The further development of such a psychology and exploration of its social and political implications is a task it behooves us to pursue.

NOTES

1. As discussed in Wachtel (1979; 1982), the reasons for this decline lie less in failings of a theoretical approach than in a failure by their proponents to take them seriously enough and carry through on their most significant features.

2. There have been vigorous challenges to the point of view I am putting forth here, and claims that in fact the neo-Freudians are shallow conformists and that it is _Freud's_ theory that is truly radical and challenging of the status quo. (See, for example, Jacoby, 1975; Lasch, 1977; Marcuse, 1955.) In part, my response to these claims can be found in a number of the chapters of _Action and Insight_ (Wachtel; 1987), but a full-scale analysis of the differing social implications of the Freudian and neo-Freudian positions is a project I hope to be able to launch before long.

3. See _The Poverty of Affluence_, Wachtel, 1983, for still other illustrations of our self-deceptions in this regard and for a psychological perspective on this state of affairs that complements Hirsch's economic perspective.

REFERENCES

Erikson, E. 1985. _Childhood and Society_. New York: W. W. Norton.

Friedman, M., and R. Friedman. 1980. _Free to Choose_. New York: Harcourt.

Habermas, J. 1971. _Knowledge and Human Interests_. Boston: Beacon.

Hirsch, F. 1976. _Social Limits to Growth_. Cambridge: Harvard University Press.

Jacoby, R. 1975. _Social Amnesia: A Critique of Conformist Psychology from Adler to Laing_. Boston: Beacon.

Lasch, C. 1977. _Haven in a Heartless World_. New York: Basic.

Marcuse, H. 1955. _Eros and Civilization_. Boston: Beacon.

Wachtel, P. L. 1979. "Karen Horney's Ironic Vision." _New Republic_, January 6, pp. 25-28.

Wachtel, P. L. 1982. Vicious Circles: The Self and the Rhetoric of Emerging and Unfolding." _Contemporary Psychoanalysis_ 18: 259-73.

Wachtel, P. L. 1983. _The Poverty of Affluence: A Psychological Portrait of the American Way of_

Life. New York: Free Press.
Wachtel, P. L. 1987. Action and Insight. New York: Guilford.

4

Proposed Values for Guiding and Evaluating Counseling and Psychotherapy

Allen E. Bergin

A survey of published and private opinions of mental health professionals revealed a previously hidden consensus concerning certain values that enhance mental health. These values concern: Freedom, Love, Identity, Truth, Universals, Symptom Management, and Work. There was disagreement about the effects of many other values on mental health.

It is argued by the author that values permeate counseling and psychotherapy, that the values of counselors and therapists should be more explicit, and that values should be openly used to guide and evaluate treatment.

It is widely agreed that values influence every phase of psychotherapy, from theories of personality and pathology, the design of change methods, and the goals of treatment, to the assessment of outcomes (Bergin, 1980a; Beutler, 1979; Graham, 1980; Rosenbaum, 1982; Wallach and Wallach, 1983). Values in this context are orienting beliefs about what is good for clients and how that good should be achieved. Value decisions affect both specific aims, such as symptom removal, and general aims, such as lifestyle changes. It is the thesis of this chapter that since values are necessarily embedded in the treatment process, they should be made explicit and should be openly used to guide and evaluate change.

There is currently, however, only a limited consensus about which values to endorse. Disagreements arise because of differences in theoretical orientation; personal philosophy; religion; and cultural, ethnic, or national background (Bergin, 1983; Sue, 1983; Strupp and Hadley, 1977). Although there is a trend in Western nations toward distinctly humanistic and naturalistic therapeutic philosophies consistent with the scientific secularism that dominates Western education, a strong countertrend exists within more theistic and conservative communities. Even secular society, however, is showing a strong trend toward reconsidering spiritual perspectives, as evidenced in part by renewed attention to various philosophies and religions (Bergin, 1980a).

Given the great diversity of value positions within both the secular and spiritual orientations, there now exists a wide array of value themes that can and do influence the thinking of psychotherapists. This diversity has led many professionals to avow a belief in ethical relativism. Such a position, however, is fraught with logical inconsistencies (Kitchener, 1980a, 1980b; Bergin 1980a, 1980b, 1980c). It is difficult to square with the notion that there are lawful behavioral consequences of one's actions. While cultural relativism clearly exists, that is; cultures differ in values; ethical relativism does not follow from this fact. The values of differing cultures are not equally healthy (Maslow, 1971).

In an attempt to achieve some coherence in this domain, I synthesized a set of values rooted in Judeo-Christian traditions that I felt were related to mental health and social integration (Bergin, 1980a). My intent was to clarify and make explicit my own views as well as values implicit in the writings of other professionals and to contrast them with some of the values common in the clinical literature.

My outline included such values as self-control; commitment to marriage, family life, and fidelity; forgiveness as an aid in psychological healing; acceptance of guilt, suffering, contrition, and restitution when one's behavior has harmed others; love and self-transcendence or self-sacrifice, as opposed to a sole focus upon self-actualization; the importance of spiritual knowledge, and so on.

I also proposed testable hypotheses, such as the following:

1. Communities that provide the combination of a viable belief structure and a network of loving, emotional support should manifest lower than normal rates of emotional and social pathology and physical disease.
2. Those groups that endorse high standards of impulse control should have lower than average rates of alcoholism, drug addiction, divorce,

emotional instability, and associated interpersonal difficulties.

3. A stable marriage and family life should constitute a psychologically and socially benevolent state. As the percentage of persons in a community who live in such circumstances increases, social pathologies should decrease and vice versa (Bergin, 1980a, pp. 102-3).

In response to that article, I received about 1,000 requests for reprints, many of which included comments about the values listed. Although the remarks showed a strong divergence of opinion about the theistic and spiritual themes (Ellis, 1980; Walls, 1980), they also showed surprising support for many of the core values I had proposed.

Excerpts from some of these positive responses (views rarely expressed in professional publications) show the importance of a viewpoint to be presented later that may otherwise seem inconsistent with professional opinion. They are represented by the following sample of extracts from letters, which are quoted with the permission of the writers.

> Ellen Berscheid, Professor of Psychology, University of Minnesota: I congratulate you for saying what I believe has needed to be said for a long time . . . . I very much hope that this paper will, in retrospect, be considered one of the most important to have been published in the area in the new decade.

> Ted Lorie, Health Services, R & D Service, Veterans Administration, Washington, D.C.: I think this is a landmark article that says several things that many people must have been thinking for years. You have done us all a great service.

> Lise Wallach, Lecturer, Department of Psychology, Duke University: [I] am extremely sympathetic with the hypotheses you describe.

> Karl Menninger, Menninger Foundation, Topeka, Kansas: I commend you on your excellent article.

> Richard Jessor, Institute of Behavioral Science, University of Colorado: Although

not in agreement with much of your position, I do appreciate your bringing it clearly before psychologists. And I do share your concern for making explicit the values that necessarily underlie and guide not only psychotherapy but psychological work as a whole. That religious values are or can be among those is difficult to dispute.

Dorothy Fahs Beck, Director of Research, Family Service Association of America: I am also wondering whether you consider that maintenance of the obviously desirable value patterns that you outlined as necessarily dependent on a theistic orientation . . . . Would it perhaps be possible, using the findings of science on child development, family systems, and the like, to provide an alternate philosophic base that would still support the value positions you outlined?

Paul Vitz, Professor of Psychology, New York University: I found it important, interesting and quite heartening. I hope it receives wide circulation.

Henk Wijngaarden, former Director of Clinical Training, Free University of Amsterdam: It was a very pleasant surprise for me, and I think you are dealing here with a very important matter . . . . I recognize the taboo among psychotherapists to speak about matters of faith . . . . I always taught my students that understanding the religious dimension of your clients is necessary to be a therapeutic expert.

Hans H. Strupp, Professor of Psychology, Vanderbilt University: On the whole, I am very much in agreement although we may differ on some aspects . . . . Major values in human relations are woven into various religious systems, and they seem to be universally true regardless of what a therapist's attitude toward a Supreme Being might be.

Robert Sears, Professor of Psychology, Stanford University: I enjoyed your article thoroughly. With your memories of 20 years ago, unrefreshed by more recent contact with me, you will be surprised to know that I agreed heartily with most of what you said. That is, I agree that for the therapist it is important to have his values as explicit as possible and the patient's values should also be explicit . . . . In some places you seem to be talking theism versus atheism. In others, there is some implication of more specific "good and bad" principles . . . . In this connection, let me tell you a quick story. In the 1930's, no instructor in psychology could avoid being an amateur psychotherapist for university students. There were no psychiatrists, no counseling services. We all did it as just part of our university service. I suppose I spent as much as five or six hours a week doing what we would now call psychotherapy. To this day I remain proudest of my accomplishment in dealing with a young devout orthodox Jewish boy who was suffering severe conflicts about his religious role and the relation of his Jewish beliefs to some of the issues that he was having to face in classes (not mine). The satisfying outcome was that he returned to his orthodox views, without further conflict, and ultimately became a rabbi . . . . The other kinds of values seem more pertinent to me, even in research. Inescapably they enter into the ways in which questions are asked and the methods by which answers are sought . . . . I do believe that every psychological researcher should be familiar with his own value system.

Albert Bandura, Professor of Psychology, Stanford University: Whether it be the role of religious values in the science and practice of psychology, humanism, radical behaviorism, or social learning theory, such ideas touch the lives of people in the field because certain proponents were willing to state them, whatever the reactions of others might be. It is through writing such that religious values will receive greater consideration in psychotherapy.

Carl R. Rogers, Center for Studies of the Person, La Jolla, California: I don't disagree as much as you might think . . . . I do believe there is some kind of a transcendent organizing influence in the

> universe which operates in man as well. I lean toward the notion that perhaps this force is a struggling force and that we are a part of the struggle to make the universe a better place to live in . . . . My present, very tentative, view is that perhaps there is an essential person which persists through time, or even through eternity . . . . Your value system is a little too narrow to suit me, but a least it is yours . . . . I had to smile the other day when talking to Mwalimu Amara; . . . He told me that when he gets to feeling depressed, he reads some of "the gospels by Rogers." When the people around laughed at his remark, he said, "Well, this guy has been writing religious stuff for many years and it's about time that he admits it."

In addition to such comments, I was surprised by positive comments from several practicing psychoanalysts, whom I had assumed would look upon these matters from a more Freudian perspective.

In concluding this list of quotations, I refer to a comment by Gary B. Walls (1980), who published a critique of my paper on values. In a letter responding to my reply to his critique, he said;

> Although the differences among us were clearly drawn, the corresponding overlap points to the possibility of fruitful discussion among different viewpoints. The contribution of this interchange I think is to dispel the notion that dogmatic opposition and stubborn, unreflective allegiance to a given point of view is a necessary stance in order to maintain ideologically pure and self-consistent ethical systems. An open system is not necessarily ethically relativistic or neutral, but acknowledges human fallibility . . . . Although I myself do not endorse theism, I feel comfortable that if its cause is furthered in a scholarly manner . . . it will prove to be a strong positive force (along with "Positive" humanism) in the advancement of ethically sound psychotherapy practice.

Like the others, Walls feels it is important to be specific about values, to endorse constructive values, and to study the results of adopting such values. This chapter is thus a response to the stimulus, provided by his and the other letters, to develop a more explicit therapeutic value orientation. What follows is merely a beginning, and it emphasizes points of agreement rather than disagreement. I feel it is important to set aside disputes about controversial values and their origins (Bergin, 1983), which could lead to endless and unfruitful debates, and instead establish areas of agreement. We thereby provide common reference points that will stimulate further development of therapeutically relevant values and enhance both theory and practice.

This brings me to the most difficult part of this paper: outlining a set of values concerning which I believe there is a reasonable consensus among counselors and psychotherapists, even though the consensus has been hidden over the years by arguments that no common ground exists and that we can legitimately operate only upon the shifting sands of relativism.

I base this outline on my reading of the therapy and personality literature, on correspondence, on discussions at conferences with colleagues in North and South America and European countries, and on doctoral dissertation research I helped supervise (Billington, 1983; Lilienfeld, 1966; Vaughn, 1971). The outline is my personal interpretation and synthesis from these sources. In addition, I compared my outline with M. Rokeach's (1973) 18 terminal and 18 instrumental values and with E. L. Shostrom's 1966, personal orientation inventory values, resulting in further adjustment and integration.

I recognize, of course, that there may be high agreement on a value that may in fact lack validity. Nevertheless, it seems important to consider values espoused by a large proportion of professionals who systematically observe the behavior of many people.

It should also be pointed out that many important values are omitted in the discussion that follows. Values such as political freedom, equal opportunity, nondiscrimination, and freedom from poverty certainly influence mental health, but to discuss them would take us far beyond the focus of this chapter. Also omitted are numerous values about which there are continuing controversy and disagreement. Although these issues are worthy of continued exploration, such a debate could not be contained in one chapter.

In Table 4.1, 23 value statements have been clustered under 7 headings, representing my distillation of consensus values for the sources noted above.

Table 4.1
Values That Enhance Mental Health

Counselors and psychotherapists should collaborate with clients to achieve the following goals:

I. Freedom, responsibility, and self-regulation

1. Freedom of choice via improving the person's range of alternatives and capacity to act well at choice points.
2. Freedom from coercion, abuse, manipulation, and the inhibiting effects of symptoms.
3. Personal independence and autonomy.
4. Personal responsibility for one's actions and their effects on oneself and others.
5. Self-control and discipline in order to achieve or live congruently with ideals, values, principles, or goals.

II. Love and relationships

1. The capacity to give and receive love and affection. This includes caring, trust, commitment, loyalty, nurturant support, and the ability to develop fulfilling emotional and physical intimacy.
2. Effective interpersonal relationship skills, especially the capacity to resolve conflict.
3. The ability to forgive others, even those who have inflicted pathologizing experiences on oneself.
4. The ability to make restitution for negative consequences of one's influence and to forgive oneself for past mistakes.
5. Commitment to family needs and growth.
6. Fidelity and loyalty in marriage.
7. Empathic sensitivity to the feelings of others and an ability to express one's feelings accurately and constructively.
8. Effective participation in a large or small mutually supportive social network with a sense of community or group identification.

III. Identity

1. The ability to prize one's own human dignity

and self-worth as one deserving of esteem from others and oneself.
2. The ability to be introspective and reflective in order to achieve deepened self-awareness, including sharing selfknowledge with others.
3. Engagement in a continuing process of self-development or actualization of capacities.

IV. Truth

1. The ability to be honest, authentic, and open.
2. A rational view of the personal and interpersonal world, extending to a value on knowledge and truth.

V. Values

1. A belief in some set of universal values.
2. Establishment of an active, orienting set of goals derived from one's values.

VI. Symptom management

1. Ability to be flexible in order to cope with the vicissitudes of life.
2. Ability to relieve distress and symptoms by means of coping strategies for managing reality stresses and for obtaining appropriate need satisfactions.

VII. Work

1. Ability to work productively, achieve, and attain competencies.

Each of these values is stated as a positive declaration, indicating that endorsing and living according to the value is likely to enhance mental health. It is assumed, then, that assisting clients to recognize the value of such guiding constructs can aid positive change processes. This is likely to be especially relevant to counseling situations where psychopathology is not too extreme. Where pathology is severe, technical interventions that are not particularly value laden must be used to bring the client toward a more rational condition before values can be used effectively. Discussing values is a fairly cognitive process that assumes a client's capacity for self-management is relatively intact. Deep emotional conflicts or serious conditioned reactions, then, should be partially alleviated before focusing on issues of lifestyle and self-regulation.

VALUES AND LIFESTYLES

Lifestyle issues are central to this discussion. Values guide lifestyles, and lifestyles have mental health consequences, just as they have physical health consequences. This concept is analogous to the trend in behavioral medicine that has identified lifestyle variables as important correlates of medical symptoms (Matarazzo, 1982). In biological disorders, it has become more evident that broad spectrum interventions may be as efficacious as single, precise interventions. For instance, nutritional and exercise habits; consumption of alcohol, nicotine, and caffeine; and quality of air and water all have wide ranging effects and correlate with a wide variety of disorders. As these broad lifestyle matters are brought into appropriate regulation, many types of problems are prevented or disappear without specific intervention.

Similarly many values imply a frame of reference for guiding behavior and regulating lifestyle so as to prevent or ameliorate psychopathologies and thus avoid the need for an endless array of precise technical interventions. Specific interventions are, of course, essential in many instances, but prevention and amelioration through modified lifestyle is certainly preferable.

IMPLICATIONS FOR PRACTICE AND RESEARCH

A variety of values have been listed and their relevance briefly explained. It is important to examine the question of how adopting and applying them might influence practice and research. The first issue in that application is how to use values without infringing on the client's self-determination.

Therapist Values and Client Self-Determination

There is a difference of opinion about whether therapists should influence client values. No matter how much therapists may agree on what behaviors are mentally healthy, many believe it is unethical to influence clients toward specific values. This argument is based upon a traditional view, first advanced by Freud, that therapeutic treatment is a technical matter that should be kept value-free. Good technique frees clients from symptoms that inhibit their agentive capacities, permitting them to make rational life decisions on their own. The therapist makes no judgment about these life decisions but is content to provide competent professional service. This view emphasizes relieving distress as its highest value and regards moral choices as irrelevant, much as a physician might relieve a bank robber's pain from a gunshot wound without considering the morality of the robber's lifestyle.

Although this position regarding psychotherapy was virtually demolished by Perry London twenty years ago (London, 1964) and has been eroded further by numerous leading writers, such as Erich Fromm, Albert Ellis, Carl R. Rogers, and others (Kitchener, 1980a; Bergin, 1980b), it still has merit, because care must be taken to avoid negative consequences when overtly dealing with values in therapy sessions.

Clients who are in pain become easily dependent upon their therapists and are vulnerable to their influence and authority (Frank, 1973). This position can easily be abused by therapists, who may take advantage of clients for the purpose of promoting their personal value agendas. Such therapist behavior should be shunned because a client's mental health cannot be advanced by giving up autonomy. It is a very delicate matter to preserve the client's autonomy while at the same time dealing with the inevitable value issues that arise during the change process. That is probably why the most common value found in the therapeutic literature concerns enhancing the client's freedom. (See Table 4.1.)

At the same time, therapists who emphasize freedom to the exclusion of the other values listed in Table 4.1, because they wish to keep the treatment setting value-free, are taking an extreme position that is difficult to defend. Indeed, empirical studies show that therapists do not remain value-free in their verbal behavior even when they intend to do so (see Bergin, 1980a).

In the process of treating clinical disorders, inevitably they have to make important choices about how to best optimize a client's functioning. It is at these decision points that therapists and clients must collaborate on arriving at goals that will facilitate change. The professional values that underlie such choices are often implicit because they are buried in theories and technical jargon. Also, we are usually not trained to elicit and help clarify client values.

It is vital that we be more explicit about values, since we use them, however unconsciously, as a means of therapeutic change. Although we may have been hesitant about this for fear of becoming manipulators of morals, being explicit actually protects clients. The more subtle our values, the more likely we are to be hidden persuaders. The more open we are about our views, the more choice clients will have in electing to be influenced or not be influenced.

Even trying to avoid a particular value choice by being noncommittal amounts to taking a value position. Our silence, for example, may be seen as consent for a particular line of action. Behavior therapy and other active therapies have made it clearer than ever before that as therapeutic agents we try to influence people in certain directions that we value and that we believe will benefit the client or others involved (Begelman, 1975).

Though we have to be patient while people struggle with their choices and may have to watch them make bad decisions without interference, it is irresponsible to fail to inform them of our educated opinions about the alternatives. Like good teachers or parents, we should at times instruct carefully. We need to be honest and open about our views, collaborate with the client in setting goals that fit his or her needs, then step aside and allow the person to exercise autonomy and face consequences. Our expertise, therefore, should help shape the goals of treatment according to our best judgment of how the disorder can most effectively be modified and how the change can best be maintained. To do less than this is to pretend we don't care about the outcome or to expend effort in behalf of goals we do not value, which is self-defeating.

Enhancing Freedom

Clients would not be clients if they had not already lost a measure of autonomy. Enhancing their capacity for agentive choice and self-regulation is therefore a major, if not <u>the</u> major, goal of professional assistance. Clients are, however, frequently like children in that their disturbances make them vulnerable and dependent upon the benevolent care of a stronger person. A client is unlikely to become fully functioning without passing through a critical period of reliance upon the therapist's support and guidance. This dependency must, of course, be temporary, and it must be used in the service of ultimate independence. It is comparable to the psychoanalytic concept of "regression in the service of the ego," a notion supported by reports showing that a child cannot become a fully functioning, autonomous adult without first passing through a period of deep trust and dependence upon a nurturant figure (Erikson, 1963).

Regardless of what kind of therapy is employed and whether acknowledged, this dependency process occurs. It is a natural, socially pervasive process of which therapists should not be afraid. During this phase two things are happening: symptoms are being alleviated and new insights or cognitive controls are taking over the person's attitudes, values, and lifestyle. These are inevitable processes that cannot be stemmed by the therapist's retreating into "techniques" or a laissez-faire relativism. They are normal processes to be used wisely and carefully. No better comparison can be made than to that of good parenting--trust is established; guided growth is stimulated; values are conveyed in a gentle, loving, and respectful way; the person being influenced becomes stronger, more assertive, and independent; the person learns ways of clarifying and testing value and lifestyle choices; the influencer decreases dependency, nurturance, and external advice, though continuing to be available with such resources, while the person experiments with new behaviors and ideas until becoming a mature and autonomous identity. This process in a client-therapist relationship makes symptomatic changes enduring and allows for future growth, adaptation, and change.

The concept being offered as the "freedom value," then, is that therapy may be construed as a method of enhancing a person's freedom or range of alternatives at a choice point. We achieve this in part by eliminating symptoms and in part by assisting with value-based cognitive reconstructions.

If we endorse a value such as enhancing freedom of choice, train therapists in such thinking, and help clients understand that we are aiming at their general capacity to choose and to act in behalf of those choices, the psychotherapy situation is put in a very broad context. We no longer are promoting to a greater good the liberation of a personality from inhibiting and distressing effects and the formation of new internal guidance mechanisms.

The therapist's temporary ascendancy is thus in the service of the client's becoming an autonomous, fully functioning person. The client then becomes able to consider a range of alternatives for optimal fulfillment at any choice point. Although this is not a new idea (see Rogers, 1961), construing it this way broadens our perspective and puts the psychotherapy situation in the context of an effort to activate people's agentive capacities to an optimal level.

Love, Relationships, and Fidelity

This is perhaps one of the most important dimensions in all of psychology. We can see its influence particularly in child rearing and in psychotherapy. As counselors and therapists, we often see the destructive effects of the absence of love and the harmful influence of isolation, deprivation, humiliation, rejection, punishment, and abuse. Indeed, parents' incapacity to love may be the single most pervasive pathologizing factor in human psychology. If we consider the source of depressions, anxieties, phobias, obsessions, family conflict, schizoid withdrawal, sexual dysfunctions, and so on; we easily conclude that hateful, punitive actions, even momentary or sporadic, can profoundly affect the developing person.

We are also well aware of the importance of a caring, nurturing quality in our behavior as psychotherapists, which, as Rogers has so well outlined, can be a powerful therapeutic antidote for such experiences (1957). It is caring about our clients that sets the stage for reforming personality, restoring ego strength, and increasing capacity to function interpersonally. Of equal importance is the power of teaching, training, and otherwise assisting the client in learning to become a loving person despite having been a victim of early abusive experiences.

Just how to implement the value of love in a therapeutic situation, however, is not always easy. In many marital conflict situations, for example, love brought the couple together but conflicts occur that erode that love. The question becomes how to reintroduce love to help resolve the conflicts. We might consider that love demands a certain amount of self-sacrifice and thus might teach a client how to extend love to a spouse in the face of hostility, pettiness, or disloyalty (Erikson, 1963). Encouraging a client to exercise such self-control, denying his or her own needs for a time, may prove to be powerfully therapeutic in the long run. The eventual quality of the couple's capacity to love might increase dramatically if self-sacrifice is effective in conveying to the partner a sense of deep loyalty and commitment, despite the partner's weakness and difficulties.

Discussion of this kind of commitment arose in relation to the question of marital fidelity at the International Conference on Psychotherapy in Bogotá, Colombia, where portions of this chapter were delivered. At a luncheon following my presentation, in which I argued that there were moral absolutes, Sol L. Garfield was asked by a participant whether he believed there are absolutes. He said he believed in "moderation in all things," with the exception of fidelity, which he said he considered absolute. Phillip C. Kendall, of the University of Minnesota, then related that he was gratified to hear our views because he and his wife had held to the same position despite nearly universal rejection of the idea by young friends with whom they were associated in the 1970s.

Discussions with many other people have revealed a hidden professional consensus on this issue that has been obscured by the popular writings of a few authors whose books have been widely quoted. Also, a pilot values survey by Jay P. Jensen (1984) showed that about three-fourths of nearly 100 mental health professionals in the Seattle area endorse fidelity.

While it is new to argue this position, it also is not routine to train new therapists to think in such value-laden terms. Helping them learn the skill of instructing their clients in ways of thinking about values and showing clients that there are connections between values and mental health consequences is a substantial innovation. Considering values helps both therapist and client to think about treatment outcomes in the broad terms of modifying lifestyle rather than in the usual short, narrow terms of simple relief from distress or symptom removal.

Universals Versus Relativism

Strupp's comment earlier in this paper that "major values . . . seem to be universally true regardless of what a therapist's attitude toward a Supreme Being might be" has been echoed by many others. Abraham H. Maslow was among the strongest advocates of such a view. He declared that "instead of cultural relativity, I am implying that there are basic underlying human standards that are cross cultural--psychologists who advocate moral and cultural relativism are not coming to grips with the real problem." (Cited in Goble, 1971, p. 92.)

Ethical relativism is not consistent with the idea that there are laws of human behavior (Kitchener, 1980b). Human growth is, thus, likely regulated in part by moral principles comparable in exactness with physical or biological laws, a position adeptly argued by Campbell (1975).

Some writers, however, object to this thesis on the grounds that its absolutist tendencies are tainted by an authoritarian, narrow and judgmental frame of reference that is incompatible with personal freedom (Ellis, 1980; Walls, 1980). This dichotomizing of lawfulness and freedom is, however, oversimplified. Obedience to moral law is, in principle, no different from obedience to physical laws. We are free to launch a space shuttle into orbit only as we precisely obey the natural principles that make it possible. It may be that behavioral laws are just as precise and obedience to them just as essential to obtaining desirable and predictable consequences. The freedom to self-actualize, for example, is predicated on obedience to the laws by which self-actualization is possible. Thus, the thinking that pits conformity to moral law against individual freedom, and then repudiates all favorable references to ethical universals, is inconsistent and misleading (Paraphrased from Bergin, 1980b).

If we take seriously the probable existence of universals, as a large proportion of clinical thinkers do, then the importance of guiding constructs for orienting one's choices and goals becomes more evident. It appears that the laws pertinent to how we should live have much to do with the way we construe the world, the way we activate our agentive capacities, and the responsibility we take for the ways in which we act.

Such patterns of cognitive evaluation and choosing we observe regularly in our clients as we discern the causes of their pain and suffering, as well as the changes that bring relief and hope. Our awareness that certain principles underlie the processes of disturbance and therapeutic improvement anchors the way we think about therapy and the way we influence clients' views about how they might regulate their lives. This, then, provides them with cognitive structures for organizing the behavior being suggested by the therapist.

A good example of the application of the concept of universals is in therapeutic attempts to promote self-control. Enhancing self-control of impulses or addictions is critical in modern practice. Such self-regulation must be guided by beliefs that the regulation is valuable, that it leads to long-term consequences beneficial to the client and to those who are important to the client. In this respect, the therapist is in the role of a teacher or instructor who is trying to help the client reconstruct the world and incorporate in the new construct system values concerning intrapsychic and interpersonal consequences of behavior.

Endorsing such values and making them explicit helps both the therapist and the client to realize that self-control can be guided in terms of possible universal themes. Self-discipline can never be optimally successful unless a commitment is made to values, and that commitment can be stronger and more lasting if the client feels he or she is committing to something that is lawful and moral, not just because somebody said so, but because it is built into the universe and is part of our nature.

RESEARCH AND THEORY

Empirical Studies of Values, Lifestyles, and Mental Health

This chapter is conceptual in nature and must be considered as a set of educated hypotheses. Much empirical work is needed to explore the implications suggested by them. Several studies are under way that test the questions raised here. Jay P. Jensen (1984), for instance, who prepared a doctoral dissertation under my supervision that involves a national survey of mental health professionals to determine their opinions about the values in Table 4.1 and a number of other values. We are also doing a longitudinal study of lifestyles that examines relationships between values and mental health. Pertinent completed studies done by others are also being reviewed. It is clear that careful, unbiased studies are needed to move forward in this area.

Cognitive Theory and Values Research

An integral feature of the cognitive revolution that is sweeping through the therapeutic scene is the notion that the ways in which people construe their experience are powerful mediators of the quality of their adjustment. Since values are cognitive constructs, they lend themselves to the same types of inquiries as other cognition and can be researched in the same way.

The works of Aaron T. Beck (1976), Ellis (1973), A. Bandura (1982), and many others have been exemplary in facilitating work in this area, though George Kelly's psychology of personal constructs long preceded the modern work and is still the most elegant of the cognitive theories (Kelly, 1955; Leitner, 1981). The proposals in this chapter fit well in these cognitive trends and should be further examined within that context, while also recognizing that cognition clearly is not the only important feature of pathology, therapeutic change, or values.

Measurement Studies

Another important potential of values research involves developing measurement techniques for assessing values specifically pertinent to mental health. A mental health values inventory would provide a means of operationalizing definitions and conceptions of mental health in new ways. We could then estimate where a person stands on such variables. We would then also have a presumably valid means of estimating changes in values. This could assist assessment before and after therapy. The former would help us diagnose the client, and the latter would help us estimate the effectiveness of therapy in relation to the kind of lifestyle dimensions that might make changes lasting. A preliminary measurement enterprise along such lines is now being explored by our research group. The evaluation of therapeutic outcomes could thus be markedly affected. We might find, for instance, that symptoms improve while the person's lifestyle simultaneously becomes negative in some respect. For instance, some reports indicate that sex therapy may improve a person's sexual performance but also deteriorate his or her relationship if special attention is not given to the kind of lifestyle values outlined here.

Values Research and Theory as a Major Trend

There have been numerous additional efforts in theory and research that have significant implication for therapeutic practices that explicitly address issues of values. Without attempting to list a comprehensive bibliography, the following are noted as a sample of important works that might be pursued further. These illustrate a major trend in the literature.

Seymor C. Post's book Moral Values and the Super Ego Concept in Psychoanalysis (1972), as well as R. Lovinger's Working with Religious Issues in Therapy (1984) and the article "Values and the Psychotherapist" by O. A. Will, Jr. (1981) provide a useful introduction to psychodynamic perspectives on values matters. London's Modes and Morals of Psychotherapy (1964) provides a classic, penetrating view of therapists as promoters of values, while C. Marshall Lowe's treatise (1976) shows just how pervasive such phenomena are. The 1979 Nebraska Symposium on Motivation (Howe and Page, 1980) concerned theory, research, and measurement of beliefs, attitudes and values; a book entitled Ethics and Values in Psychotherapy: A Guidebook, edited by Max Rosenbaum (1982), addresses values issues in the context of practice; a book entitled Exploring Human Values: Psychological and Philosophical Considerations by Kalish and Collier (1981), deals with many conceptual issues; and a 1980 special issue of the journal Psychotherapy (Graham, 1980) dealt entirely with values. The writings of Thomas S. Szasz also provide provocative reading on these topics (Szasz, 1974, 1978; Szasz and Nemiroff, 1963). Other important sources include P. Kessel and J. F. McBrearty (1967); M. M. Vardy and S. R. Kay (1982); and J. A. Khan and D. G. Cross (1983; 1984).

These authors and editors are struggling with the same issues discussed in this chapter. They suggest that values have an undergirding and over-arching influence on our field, an influence of which we have sometimes been deliberately ignorant.

CONCLUSION

Readers may not agree with all I have asserted here, but the points discussed are eminently subject to definition, description, measurement, research, and testing. I hope further examination will occur and that it will provoke us to reconsider the gravity of what we do when we try to influence a human life.

Obviously, the present effort provides only a beachhead in a territory yet to be fully explored. Dozens of values have not been mentioned that may have strong implication for healthy functioning. The fact that psychotherapy, as we know it, has been formulated mainly in the secular centers of Western Europe and North America induces a cultural narrowness about values and mental health that will have to be broadened as this work continues. Nevertheless, we have to begin somewhere with the best estimates we have as to which values lead to which consequences.

When we reconstrue the psychotherapist's role partly as one of evaluating and guiding value decisions, we therefore have to do so tentatively and with an awareness that we are entering a sensitive domain. But it is a domain through which I believe we are likely to have a more positive and lasting influence. In effect, this means bringing values into our traditional empirical and rational framework so that the essential variables that are reflected in value dimensions can be integrated within the traditional scientific modes to which we are already dedicated. Despite the imperfections and struggles we must deal with in such a challenging task, the possible results provide considerable incentive. Hopefully, many persons of diverse persuasions and backgrounds will collaborate in progressing towards this higher synthesis.

REFERENCES

Bandura, A. 1982. "Self-Efficacy Mechanism in Human Agency." American Psychologist, 37: 122-47.

Beck, A. T. 1976. Cognitive Therapy and the Emotional Disorders. New York: International Universities Press.

Begelman, D. A. 1975. "Ethical and Legal Issues of Behavior Modification." In M. Hersen, R. M. Eisler, and R. M. Miller, Eds. Progress in Behavior Modification. New York: Academic Press, vol. 1, pp. 159-89).

Bergin, A. E. 1980a. "Psychotherapy and Religious Values." Journal of Consulting and Clinical Psychology, 48: 95-105.

Bergin, A. E. 1980b. "Religious and Humanistic

Values: A Reply to Ellis and Walls." Journal of Consulting and Clinical Psychology, 48: 642-45.
Bergin, A. E. 1980c. "Behavior Therapy and Ethical Relativism: Time for Clarity." Journal of Consulting and Clinical Psychology, 48: 11-13.
Bergin, A. E. 1983. "Religiosity and Mental Health: A Critical Re-evaluation and Meta-analysis." Professional Psychology, 14: 170-84.
Beutler, L. 1979. "Values, Beliefs, Religion and the Persuasive Influence of Psychotherapy." Psychotherapy: Theory, Research and Practice, 16: 432-40.
Billington, L. 1983. "Psychotherapy Outcome as a Function of Client-Therapist Values Relationships and Client Values Change." Ph.D. diss. Fuller Theological Seminary, Pasadena, Calif.
Campbell, D. T. 1975. "On the Conflicts between Biological and Social Evolution and between Psychology and Moral Tradition." American Psychologist, 30: 1103-20.
Cross, D. G., and J. A. Khan. 1983. "The Values of Three Practitioner Groups: Religious and Moral Aspects." Counseling and Values, 28: 13-19.
Ellis, A. 1973. Humanistic Psychotherapy: The Rational-Emotive Approach. New York: Crown.
Ellis, A. 1980. "Psychotherapy and Atheistic Values: A Response to A. E. Bergin's 'Psychotherapy and Religious Values'." Journal of Consulting and Clinical Psychology, 48: 635-39.
Erikson, E. H. 1963. Childhood and Society. 2nd ed. New York: Norton.
Frank, J. D. 1973. Persuasion and Healing. Baltimore: Johns Hopkins University Press.
Goble, F. G. 1971. The Third Force: The Psychology of Abraham Maslow. New York: Pocket Books.
Graham, S. R., ed. 1980. "Values in Psychotherapy." Psychotherapy: Theory, Research and Practice, 17: no. 4: special issue.
Howe, H. E., and M. M. Page, eds. Nebraska Symposium on Motivation, 1979. Lincoln, University of Nebraska Press.
Jensen, J. P. 1984. "Mental Health Values of Professional Therapists: A National Interdisciplinary Survey." Unpublished pilot data, Brigham Young University, Psychology Department, Provo, Utah.
Kalish, R. A., and K. W. Collier. 1981. Exploring

Human Values: Psychological and Philosophical Considerations. Monterey, Calif.: Brooks/Cole.
Kelly, G. A. 1955. The Psychology of Personal Constructs. Vols. 1-2. New York: Norton.
Kessel, P., and McBrearty, J. F. 1967. "Values and Psychotherapy: A Review of the Literature." Perceptual and Motor Skills, 25: 669-90.
Khan, J. A., and D. G. Cross. 1983. "Mental Health Professionals: How Different Are Their Values?" American Mental Health Counselors Association Journal, 6: 42-51.
Khan, J. A., and D. G. Cross. 1984. "Mental Health Professional and Client Values: Similar or Different?" Australian Journal of Sex, Marriage, & Family, 4: 71-78.
Kitchener, R. F. 1980a. "Ethical Relativism and Behavior Therapy." Journal of Consulting and Clinical Psychology, 48: 1-7.
Kitchener, R. F. 1980b. "Ethical Relativism, Ethical Naturalism, and Behavior Therapy. Journal of Consulting and Clinical Psychology, 48: 14-16.
Leitner, L. M. 1981. "Psychopathology and the Differentiation of Values, Emotions and Behaviors: A Repertory Grid Study." British Journal of Psychiatry, 138: 147-53.
Lilienfeld, D. M. 1966. "The Relationship between Mental Health Information and Moral Values of Lower Class Psychiatric Clinic Patients and Psychiatric Evaluation and Disposition." Ph.D. diss. Columbia University, New York, N.Y. Dissertation Abstracts, 27: 610B-611B.
London, P. 1964. The Modes and Morals of Psychotherapy. New York: Holt, Rinehart & Winston.
Lovinger, R. 1984. Working with Religious Issues in Therapy. New York: Macmillan.
Lowe, C. M. 1976. Value Orientations in Counseling and Psychotherapy: The Meanings of Mental Health. 2nd ed. Cranston, R.I.: Carroll.
Maslow, A. H. 1971. The Farther Reaches of Human Nature. New York: Viking.
Matarazzo, J. D. 1982. "Behavioral Health's Challenge to Academic, Scientific, and Professional Psychology." American Psychologist, 37: 1-14.
Post, S. C., ed. 1972. Moral Values and the Superego Concept in Psychoanalysis. New York: International Universities Press.
Rogers, C. R. 1957. "The Necessary and Sufficient Conditions of Therapeutic Personality Change." Journal of Consulting Psychology, 22: 95-103.

Rogers, C. R. 1961. Becoming a Person. Boston: Houghton Mifflin.
Rokeach, M. 1973. The Nature of Human Values. New York: Free Press.
Rosenbaum, M., ed. 1982. Ethics and Values in Psychotherapy: A Guidebook. New York: Free Press.
Shostrom, E. L. 1966. Personal Orientation Inventory Manual. San Diego: Educational and Industrial Testing Service.
Strupp, H. H., and S. M. Hadley. 1977. "A Tripartite Model of Mental Health and Therapeutic Outcomes." American Psychologist 32: 187-96.
Sue, S. 1983. "Ethnic Minority Issues in Psychology." American Psychologist, 38: 583-92.
Szasz, T. S. 1974. The Myth of Mental Illness. Rev. ed. New York: Harper and Row.
Szasz, T. S. 1978. The Myth of Psychotherapy: Mental Healing as Religion, Rhetoric and Repression. Garden City, N.Y.: Doubleday.
Szasz, T. S., and R. A. Nemiroff. 1963. "A Questionnaire Study of Psychoanalytic Practices and Opinions." Journal of Nervous and Mental Disease, 137: 209-21.
Vardy, M. M., and S. R. Kay. The Therapeutic Value of Psychotherapists' Values and Therapy Orientations." Psychiatry, 45: 226-33.
Vaughn, J. L. 1971. "Measurement and Analysis of Values Pertaining to Psychotherapy and Mental Health." Ph.D. diss. Columbia University, New York, N.Y., 1971. Dissertation Abstracts International, 32: 3655B-56B.
Wallach, M. A., and L. Wallach. 1983. Psychology's Sanction for Selfishness. San Francisco: Freeman.
Walls, G. B. 1980. "Values and Psychotherapy: A Comment on 'Psychotherapy and religious values'. Journal of Consulting and Clinical Psychology, 48: 640-41.
Will, O. A., Jr. 1981. "Values and the Psychotherapist." American Journal of Psychoanalysis, 41: 203, 210.

PART II

NEW THEORETICAL TRENDS IN PSYCHOTHERAPY

5

Common and Specific Factors in Cognitive Therapy

Diane B. Arnkoff

This chapter presents the similarities and differences between cognitive therapy and other contemporary forms of therapy. I will use the term "cognitive therapy" throughout, but I am not restricting my discussion to any one particular theorist. For the purposes of this chapter, I will define cognitive therapy as a therapy that is cognitive in its theory of psychopathology and behavior change. More specifically, cognitive therapy as it is currently practiced can be defined by the following characteristics:

1. The theory of the therapy describes the development of adaptive and maladaptive behavior in terms of cognitive processes (D. Arnkoff and G. V. Glass, 1982; Beck, 1976);
2. The therapist sees the therapeutic endeavor as a collaborative educational process;
3. The therapist makes use of various procedures, frequently, though certainly not exclusively, those called cognitive and behavioral;
4. The therapy is usually relatively short in duration;
5. The theory of the therapy seeks to explain change in therapy primarily as a cognitive process (Arnkoff, 1980; Arnkoff & Glass, 1982; Goldfried, 1979; Mahoney, 1974; Meichenbaum, 1977; Merluzzi, et al., 1981); and
6. The therapist is committed to a scholarly examination of theories and procedures, including empirical tests.

The therapies that clearly fall under the definition are Aaron Beck's cognitive therapy (Beck

1976; Beck, et al., 1979), rational-emotive therapy or RET (Ellis, 1962; Ellis & Grieger, 1977), and those forms of cognitive-behavior therapy or cognitive-behavior modification that emphasize cognitive processes (e.g., Kendall and Hollon, 1979; Meichenbaum, 1977).

Several theorists of psychotherapy process have argued that common factors operate in virtually all therapies (e.g., Frank, 1973; Garfield, 1980; Goldfried, 1980; Strupp, 1977). The common factors form the structure of all therapies, and they certainly play a large role in cognitive therapy, as in other therapies. The content of cognitive therapy, however, is distinct from that of other therapies. It is an empirical question as to whether this specific content affects outcome over and above the common factors (Kazdin and Wilcoxon, 1976). Following from this distinction between common and specific factors, I will describe several components of cognitive therapy. In some respects, each component seems to operate in cognitive therapy in a manner consistent with all therapies; I will call these aspects the common factors. In other respects, however, cognitive therapy differs on each component from at least some other forms of therapy. I will call these differences the specific factors. It must be emphasized that empirical evaluation of any unique contribution of these specific factors is essential, but has yet to be undertaken.

The following aspects of cognitive therapy will be discussed:

1. The establishment of a constructive therapeutic relationship;
2. The therapist as a model of adaptive adjustment;
3. The therapeutic interaction as a source of information for the therapist;
4. The therapeutic rationale in cognitive therapy; and
5. The cognitive and behavioral methods often used in cognitive therapy.

THE ESTABLISHMENT OF A CONSTRUCTIVE RELATIONSHIP

The Relationship as a Common Factor

Hans H. Strupp (1977) has noted that in as much as technique is important, psychotherapy is not wholly dependent on the therapist for its effect;

however, the therapist's personality and manner are by no means irrelevant. In cognitive therapy, as in any other therapy, one of the therapist's most important tasks is to foster and sustain a constructive relationship with the client. In a treatment like cognitive therapy, with its emphasis on various strategies, it may be easy to lose sight of the crucial role played by the relationship. As Aaron T. Beck and others (1979) point out, the inexperienced therapist may become enamored of techniques and forget to put effort into the relationship, which is the foundation for the effectiveness of the techniques.

Much discussion in the psychotherapy literature has centered on what constitutes a constructive relationship in therapy. A useful way of defining the constructive relationship is to see it as a relationship in which the client is prepared to be influenced by the therapist.

Expectations of therapeutic success may play an important role in this influence process. In his discussion of expectations in therapy, G. T. Wilson (1980) reviewed research on the influence of both outcome and self-efficacy expectations (A. Bandura, 1977) in treatment for fear reduction. Extrapolating from his review, expectations may play a role in determining therapy success by the following sequence: The client's faith in the therapist, which is fostered by the relationship leads to an increase in the client's expectations of a positive outcome from therapy. These increased outcome expectations, in turn, persuade the client to follow the therapist's lead in trying out new behaviors. Bandura has found empirical support for his hypothesis that such behavior change increases self-efficacy expectations, that is, the expectations of personal capability (A. Bandura, 1977; Bandura and Adams, 1977). Increased self-efficacy expectations, in turn, influence maintenance of the behavior change (Wilson, 1980).

Therapeutic influence through the creation of a positive therapeutic relationship may, thus, affect the client through such means as raising expectations for change. A familiar question arises here: What is required on the part of the therapist for this constructive relationship to be formed? To date, no empirical investigations of this essential question have been undertaken in cognitive therapy. D. E. Orlinsky and K. I. Howard's (1978) conclusion from their review of process-outcome studies was that good outcome tends to be associated with certain attitudes and behaviors from the therapist:

active and positive task behavior, warmth, and respect. No such studies have been undertaken with cognitive therapy. It would be most interesting to see if such behaviors were also generally associated with positive outcome in cognitive therapy.

The Relationship as a Specific Factor

In cognitive therapy, a particular kind of therapeutic alliance is formed, one that is collaborative and educational. Because the therapy stresses the rapid development of client competency to continue the therapeutic procedures after termination, the therapy can be short, and maintenance of therapeutic gains is intended to be enhanced.

Collaboration in cognitive therapy means that the therapy is a joint effort between the therapist and client against the client's problem (Beck, 1976). Explicit consensus is sought on the nature of the client's problem, the goals of therapy, and how the goals are to be reached. Beck (1976) advises the cognitive therapist to be careful to attend to the client's agenda, including how this agenda changes from session to session. The emphasis in the collaboration is on solving problems, not on pathology in the client. Such collaboration probably enhances the congruence of therapist-client expectations for therapy, which has been found to be related to remaining in therapy (Garfield, 1978; Parloff, et al., 1978).

Clearly, collaboration in therapy does not mean equal roles for therapist and client. The therapist is the leader but trains the client for leadership. Several specific procedures in therapy aim at ensuring this collaboration. The client's goals for therapy are assessed early and also at each session. The therapist carefully explains the cognitive point of view on the meaning of maladaptive behavior and gives the rationale for all therapeutic procedures, sometimes citing research evidence in terms the client can understand. Beck and others (1979) advise obtaining the client's reactions to each session at the end, looking especially for negative reactions. Finally, homework assignments such as monitoring of thoughts are jointly designed. Clients are progressively encouraged to take more control as they learn the therapeutic rationale and procedures.

Cognitive therapy is educational as well as collaborative. The emphasis is on learning rather than on being cured. The therapist explicitly teaches the cognitive rationale that some of the client's assumptions or beliefs are dysfunctional. The therapist also teaches techniques to modify these beliefs, such as monitoring of automatic thoughts, or self-statements, examination of evidence, and carrying out of experiments to test assumptions. The cognitive therapist teaches the client to be a personal scientist (Kelly, 1955). The ultimate goal of cognitive therapy is to teach clients how to use these change methods themselves; the process of therapy is "learning to learn" (Beck, 1976).

It is important in cognitive therapy, and perhaps in all therapies, for the client to view the process of change as self-determined. M. R. Goldfried and G. C. Davison (1976) conclude from a review of the attitude change literature that persuasion will be maximized if clients themselves state arguments to refute their dysfunctional beliefs instead of hearing the arguments from another person. Several studies on obesity and insomnia have also shown that maintenance of behavior change is increased if the client attributes the change to his or her own actions rather than to an external agent such as the therapist or a drug (e.g., Davison and Valins, 1969; Jeffrey, 1974). Although cognitive therapy is an educational process, self-discovery and learning of tools for self-change are emphasized. It is likely that the client's sense of self-determination increases as cognitive therapy progresses. Toward the end of therapy, the client takes more responsibility for discovering assumptions, offering arguments and evidence against them, and designing behavior change experiments.

Among cognitive therapists, some differences can be found in teaching style. Beck and others (1979) emphasize that it is important not to force the teaching on the client. Albert Ellis, (1962), on the other hand, is usually more didactic than Beck and, in fact, more argumentive than most other cognitive therapists. It is not uncommon, for example, for Ellis to assert bluntly to clients that they are thinking irrationally. Such confrontation does not indicate a poor relationship. Ellis also maintains that acceptance of the client (though not of the client's irrational beliefs) is essential, and his style is not incompatible with good rapport with the client.

The importance for clients to attribute change to themselves was discussed earlier. On this basis,

Ellis's style is thought by some to be less effective than a style requiring the client to take more of the lead. However, the stage of therapy may be an important factor here. If a therapist adopting Ellis's vigorous style early in therapy has also encouraged the client to take more responsibility for directing the work once he or she has learned the rationale and methods of RET, the final results may well be the desired self-attribution for change. This question of therapist style in cognitive therapy and client self-persuasion is worthy of empirical study. Therapist style could be assessed both by ratings of behaviors such as information giving and by measures of activity such as frequency and length of interventions at different stages of therapy.

THE THERAPIST AS A MODEL FOR ADAPTIVE ADJUSTMENT

Modeling as a Common Factor

One function of the therapeutic relationship may be to establish the therapist as a model. In all therapies, the therapist becomes a model for the client of adaptive behavior, whether or not such modeling is planned by the therapist (Garfield, 1980). In the client's demoralized state (Frank, 1976), he or she may lack adequate role models. As the therapist persuades the client of the therapeutic procedures, he or she also educates the client as to the other aspects of the therapist's behavior, such as how the therapist responds to problems that come up in therapy.

In an active therapy like cognitive therapy, the therapist displays a great deal of problem-solving behavior that the client could adopt. Providing such problem-solving by the therapist is adaptive, and cognitive therapy may be particularly strong in this common factor (along with other active therapies like behavior therapy). The emphasis here is not on activity level per se; activity level alone does not necessarily make for better outcome (Pope, 1977). Rather, the emphasis here on activity level relates to the degree and specificity of information available to the client, which may be associated with better outcome.

Modeling as a Specific Factor

In cognitive therapy, the therapist models

optimism about the client's ability to change. The advantages are demonstrated of maintaining positively toned emotions even when reality would be just as consistent with pessimism, in that optimism allows for further coping, while pessimism would not. The relentless optimism of a therapist like Beck may be one reason that cognitive therapy has been shown to be effective in treating depression.

The cognitive therapist also consistently adopts a problem-solving attitude in response to therapeutic events, taking the role of the personal scientist (Kelly, 1955; Mahoney, 1977). With both appropriate humility and confidence, the therapist ideally is willing to take on whatever the client presents (Beck, 1976). Thus the client who tends to surrender to adversity would most likely benefit from adopting the problem-solving attitude displayed by the cognitive therapist.

THERAPEUTIC INTERACTIONS AS A SOURCE OF INFORMATION

Interaction as a Common Factor

Just as the client learns from modeling the therapist's behavior, so the therapist learns about the client by observing the client's functioning within the session. These observations then form the basis for therapeutic interventions.

A focus on within therapy behavior has a number of advantages that probably contribute to its effectiveness. First, it allows the therapist to obtain information on the client's functioning directly rather than through the client's report. If the client reports on behavior outside of therapy, the therapist receives the information through the (perhaps dysfunctional) perspective of the client. By observing the client directly in therapy, the therapist can put his or her own perspective on the behavior (Garfield, 1980). Second, dealing with current behavior in the session reverts the attention of both therapist and client, especially because of the emotional arousal that comes from discussing the current situation. Third, a focus on within therapy behavior allows the client the opportunity to try out new behavior with the therapist. Although the therapeutic relationship is important to the client, it does not have the longitudinal importance to the client of a relationship such as marriage. It may be easier and safer for the client to act differently with the therapist before trying it out with others. To the extent that the situation within therapy accurately recreates the client's problem and corresponding emotions, the client can make discoveries and try new behavior that will be generalizable outside therapy.

The Interaction as a Specific Factor

Cognitive therapists are alert for examples of dysfunctional thinking that occur within a session. The position of most cognitive therapists on the use of such information is that it is advantageous providing the therapist pays careful attention to the generalizability of what the client learns. One tactic often used both to allow the therapist to observe dysfunctional thinking and to pave the way for generalization is to have the client imagine or role-play a realistic problem.

The cognitive therapist also focuses on relationship issues as they seem relevant. In a similar manner to the psychodynamic therapist, the cognitive therapist views such issues as having the potential to expose and change the client's distorted perception of events. Beck and others (1979) advise being watchful for relationship issues and making them explicit when they occur. The procedure then is to examine them as any other issue in therapy is examined. Relationship issues in cognitive therapy are thought to be important both because of their disruptive power if ignored, and because they provide in vivo information that can be used therapeutically (Beck et al., 1979). However, transference issues are far more central to psychodynamic therapy than to cognitive therapy. In cognitive therapy, client distortions toward the therapist are addressed like any other distortions. Although working in vivo has advantages, the cognitive therapist uses imagery and role playing to bring issues into therapy in addition to attending to their therapist-client relationship.

The Therapeutic Rationale as a Common Factor

According to Jerome D. Frank (1973), the content of the rationale in a therapy is not as important as its comprehensiveness and prescriptive nature. "Within a broad often not fully articulated philosophy of life, the rationale of each school of psychotherapy explains the cause of the sufferer's distress, specifies desirable goals for him, and prescribes procedures for attaining them" (p. 327). Sol L. Garfield (1980) suggests that a match between client and rationale may be advantageous, in that some clients may find certain rationales more believable. The persuasiveness of the therapist, however, may be as much a factor in the client's acceptance of the rationale as the content. Frank (1973) notes that an essential condition for a successful rationale is that it takes an optimistic stand on the possibility for client change. As D. W. Johnson and R. P. Matross (1977) explain this point, the rationale must attribute the problem to an unstable cause that the client can influence.

The Therapeutic Rationale as a Specific Factor

In cognitive therapy, the therapist presents the rationale that what individuals believe colors what they feel and do. Maladaptive feelings and behaviors can be changed, according to the rationale, by modifying distorted beliefs, such as the belief of a depressed client that everyone will reject him or her. Both internal and external sources of influence on behavior are postulated, but the emphasis is on those aspects that are changeable, namely, client beliefs and actions. The rationale thus fits Frank's (1973) specification of optimism, in that change is within the power of the client. The rationale focuses on present beliefs and their ramifications rather than on the past sources of these beliefs.

There may be several aspects of the cognitive rationale that make it believable to a wide range of clients. Though the emphasis is on dysfunctional beliefs within the client, the therapy takes external influences on the client's behavior into account as well. While the rationale for therapy is readily understandable, it is not overly simplistic. Finally, the rationale not only attributes the problem to unstable causes that the client can influence, but it also says that these changes can be accomplished relatively quickly. In concert with the persuasive power of the therapist through the therapeutic relationship, these aspects of the cognitive rationale may maximize its believability.

THERAPEUTIC CHANGE PROCEDURES

Change Procedures as a Common Factor

The therapeutic rationale in every therapy prescribes certain change procedures for the client. Because of the trust the client has for the therapist, he or she is motivated to carry out the procedures.

Although the content of change procedures varies across therapies, Goldfried (1980) suggests that one common effect of these procedures is that of "providing the patient/client with new, corrective experiences" (p. 994). A related strategy may be that of disrupting ongoing patterns of experience to allow the more adaptive experiences to be substituted. The assumption here is that the client has adopted rigid, maladaptive patterns--in other words, the client has gotten into a rut. Any of several change procedures may work to disrupt the maladaptive pattern, providing the client is motivated through the relationship to try the procedures. Nevertheless, there may also be differences among clients in their susceptibility to various procedures. For example, cognitive therapy has been found to be especially effective for depression (e.g., Rush et al., 1977). One reason for its effectiveness may be that its active procedures, both behavioral and verbal, serve to interrupt the client's dysphoric affect.

Change Procedures as a Specific Factor

As explained in the introduction to this chapter, cognitive therapy is defined more by its cognitive theory than by specific change procedures that are invariably used. Certain cognitive and behavioral methods, however, are frequently employed. These include Socratic dialogue (leading questions aimed at helping clients persuade themselves of the dysfunctional nature of beliefs), identification of dysfunctional thoughts through self-monitoring homework and through exploration within the session, behavioral rehearsal, and behavioral experiments designed to test the client's assumptions (Beck et al., 1979). In keeping with the theory of therapy, the goal is cognitive change, but cognitive change does not necessarily require "cognitive" techniques (A. Bandura, 1977; Glass and Arnkoff, 1982).

Behavior change plays a special role in cognitive therapy, and perhaps in all therapies. Much of the activity of cognitive therapy, using cognitive, behavioral, and other methods, is aimed toward achieving behavior change. Albert Bandura (1977) hypothesizes that an increase in self-efficacy expectations is best attained by performance accomplishments. Similarly, Phillip C. Kendall and S. D. Hollon (1981) suggest that the self-statement "I can do it" acquires its power over behavior only if the client can believe it--that is, only if the client has performed behavior consistent with the self-statement.

Why is behavior change so important as a means of changing cognitive processes? Behavior change may play this role because it is effective in creating <u>indisputable evidence</u> of the therapist's point of view. When, for example, a client claims that everyone will reject him or her, but then at the therapist's suggestion makes a rare overture to an acquaintance and finds it is not rejected, the evidence of the behavioral act is hard to ignore. As Michael J. Mahoney (1980) has suggested, behavior that is inconsistent with prior beliefs but consistent with emerging beliefs is powerful persuasion toward the new beliefs. Cognitive change is the ultimate goal of cognitive therapy, but in many cases it may be best achieved through behavior change. A most important use of therapeutic influence, then, is to motivate the client to change behavior.

FUTURE DIRECTIONS

In this chapter, several factors have been discussed in which cognitive therapy is both similar to and different from other forms of therapy. This chapter is a first attempt at such delineation of common and specific factors in cognitive therapy. To date, no empirical research in cognitive therapy has addressed the issues discussed here.

Several lines of such research have been suggested in the course of this chapter. Therapist activity level in different states of cognitive therapy as it relates to outcome is one possible pursuit. Another is examination of the effects of different relationship building behaviors on the part of the cognitive therapist, and whether these behaviors must vary according to client factors such as disorder. The latter line of research would seem to be especially important because of its implications for training.

Although cognitive therapy currently enjoys considerable popularity, it is clear to this author that much of its effect derives from factors it shares with other therapies. The most fruitful direction may be to investigate the manner in which general change principles, including the therapeutic relationship, operate in cognitive therapy. The ultimate question in cognitive therapy, as in other therapies, is how to adapt therapeutic strategies with particular therapists and clients so that these general change principles may be maximized.

REFERENCES

Arnkoff, D. B. 1980. "Psychotherapy from the Perspective of Cognitive Theory." In M. J. Mahoney, ed. Psychotherapy Process: Current Issues and Future Directions. New York: Plenum.

Arnkoff, D. B. 1983. "Common and Specific Factors in Cognitive Therapy." In M. J. Lambert, ed. Psychotherapy and Patient Relations. Homewood, Ill.: Dorsey.

Arnkoff, D. B., and & C. R. Glass. 1982. "Clinical Cognitive Constructs: Examination, Evaluation, and Elaboration." In P. C. Kendall, ed. Advances in Cognitive-Behavioral Research and Therapy. Vol. 1. New York: Academic.

Bandura, A. 1977. "Self-Efficacy: Towards a Unifying Theory of Behavioral Change." Psychological Review, 84: 191-215.

Bandura, A., and N. E. Adams. 1977. Analysis of Self-Efficacy Theory of Behavioral Change." Cognitive Therapy and Research, 1: 287-308.

Beck, A. T. 1976. Cognitive Therapy and the Emotional Disorders. New York: International Universities Press.

Beck, A. T., A. J. Rush, B. F. Shaw, and G. Emery. 1979. Cognitive Therapy of Depression: A Treatment Manual. New York: Guilford.

Davison, G. C., and S. Valins. 1969. "Maintenance of Self-attributed and Drug-attributed Behavior Change." Journal of Personality and Social Psychology, 11: 25-33.

Ellis, A. 1962. Reason and Emotion in Psychotherapy. New York: Lyle Stuart.

Ellis, A., and R. Grieger, eds. 1977. Handbook of Rational-Emotive Therapy. New York: Springer.

Frank, J. D. 1973. Persuasion and Healing. Rev.

ed. New York: Schocken.

Frank, J. D. 1976. "Restoration of Morale and Behavior Change." In A. Burton, ed. What Makes Behavior Change Possible? New York: Brunner/Mazel.

Garfield, S. L. 1978. "Research on Client Variables in Psychotherapy." In S. L. Garfield and A. E. Bergin, eds. Handbook of Psychotherapy and Behavior Change. 2nd ed. New York: Wiley.

Garfield, S. L. 1980. Psychotherapy: An Eclectic Approach. New York: Wiley.

Glass, C. R., and D. B. Arnkoff. 1982. "Think Cognitively: Selected Issues in Cognitive Assessment and Therapy." In P. C. Kendall, ed. Advances in Cognitive-Behavioral Research and Therapy. Vol. 1. New York: Academic.

Goldfried, M. R. 1979. "Anxiety Reduction through Cognitive-Behavioral Intervention." In P. C. Kendall and S. D. Hollon, eds. Cognitive-Behavioral Interventions: Theory, Research, and Procedures. New York: Academic.

Goldfried, M. R. 1980. "Toward the Delineation of Therapeutic Change Principles." American Psychologist, 35: 991-99.

Goldfried, M. R. and G. C. Davison. 1976. Clinical Behavior Therapy. New York: Holt, Rinehart and Winston.

Jeffrey, D. B. 1974. "A Comparison of the Effects of External-Control and Self-Control on the Modification and Maintenance of Weight." Journal of Abnormal Psychology, 83: 404-10.

Johnston, D. W., and R. P. Matross. 1977. "Interpersonal Influence in Psychotherapy: A Social Psychological View." In A. S. Curman and A. M. Razin, eds. Effective Psychotherapy: A Handbook of Research. New York: Pergamon.

Kazdin, A. E., and L. A. Wilcoxon. "Systematic Desensitization and Nonspecific Treatment Effects: A Methodological Evaluation." Psychological Bulletin, 83: 729-58.

Kelly, G. A. 1955. The Psychology of Personal Constructs. New York: Norton.

Kendall, P. C., and S. D. Hollon, eds. 1979. Cognitive-Behavioral Interventions: Theory, Research, and Procedures. New York: Academic.

Kendall, P. C., and S. D. Hollon. 1981. "Assessing Self-Referent Speech: Methods in the Measurement of Self-Statements." In P. C. Kendall and S. D. Hollon, eds. Assessment Strategies for Cognitive-Behavioral Interventions. New York: Academic.

Mahoney, M. J. 1974. Cognition and Behavior Modification. Cambridge, Mass.: Ballinger.
Mahoney, M. J. 1977. "Personal Science: A Cognitive Learning Therapy." In A. Ellis and R. Grieger, eds. Handbook of Rational-Emotive Therapy. New York: Springer.
Mahoney, M. J. 1980. "Psychotherapy and the Structure of Personal Revolutions." In M. J. Mahoney, ed. Psychotherapy Process: Current Issues and Future Directions. New York: Plenum.
Meichenbaum, D. 1977. Cognitive-Behavior Modification. New York: Plenum.
Merluzzi, T. V., T. Rudy, and C. R. Glass. "The Information Processing Paradigm: Implication for Clinical Science." In T. V. Merluzzi, C. R. Glass, and M. Genest, eds. Cognitive Assessment. New York: Guilford.
Orlinsky, D. E., and K. I. Howard. 1978. "The Relation of Process to Outcome in Psychotherapy." In S. L. Garfield and A. E. Bergin, eds. Handbook of Psychotherapy and Behavior Change, 2nd ed. New York: Wiley.
Parloff, M. B., I. E. Waskow, and B. E. Wolfe. "Research on Therapist Variables in Relation to Process and Outcome." In S. L. Garfield and A. E. Bergin, eds. Handbook of Psychotherapy and Behavior Change, 2nd ed. New York: Wiley.
Pope, B. 1977. "Research on Therapeutic Style." In A. S. Gurman and A. M. Razin, eds. Effective Psychotherapy: A Handbook of Research. New York: Pergamon.
Rush, A. J., A. T. Beck, M. Kovacs, and S. D. Hollon. "Comparative Efficacy of Cognitive Therapy and Pharmacotherapy in the Treatment of Depressed Outpatients." Cognitive Therapy and Research, 1: 17-37.
Strupp, H. H. 1977. "A Reformulation of the Dynamics of the Therapist's Contribution." In A. S. Gurman and A. M. Razin, eds. Effective Psychotherapy: A Handbook of Research. New York: Pergamon.
Wilson, G. T. 1980. "Toward Specifying the 'Nonspecific' Factors in Behavior Therapy: A Social-Learning Analysis." In M. J. Mahoney, ed. Psychotherapy Process: Current Issues and Future Directions. New York: Plenum.

6

Psychotherapy: A Journey, Not a Destination, or Rogerian Psychotherapy Revisited

G. Marian Kinget

There is one statement about psychotherapy on which one can expect to find perfect consensus--perhaps the only such statement in the whole of the literature. It concerns the muddled state of the field. A state so bewilderingly diverse that the identity of psychotherapy as a profession is hardly recognizable any longer. The most heterogeneous theories and practices, some of them radically antithetical, all claim to fall under the currently prestigious umbrella of psychotherapy. R. Herrink's Psychotherapy Handbook (Herrink, 1980), now almost ten years old, lists over 250 different approaches, and proliferation continues.

The serious observer has no alternative but to conclude that, in psychotherapy, anything goes. Teachers and practitioners alike are no longer in a position to make a justification as to what brand to adopt in their work. Hence their choice is bound to amount to a random pick, since time limits prohibit them from becoming sufficiently well acquainted with enough approaches to allow for a valid choice.

There was a time when psychotherapies possessed a stated and articulate identity. Discussions and papers about the orthodoxy of certain fine points abounded, to the detriment of discussion of significant issues concerning the enterprise as a whole, though an overall examination was then already overdue.

Once the psychoanalytic monopoly was broken, the doors for psychotherapeutic initiative were flung wide open. There was, of course, ample opportunity for modification and expansion between the two leading and virtually antithetical systems. Had the pioneers who seized this opportunity presented their contributions for what they basically were (offshoots from either one of these fountainheads, enriched by bridging efforts and sometimes brilliant insights) the field as a whole might have gained in clarity, organization, and unity. Instead, each coined new, often intriguing, labels for apparently rather hastily constructed systems. The ambitious professional felt compelled to devise some new formula and to bolster it with publications proclaiming therapeutic virtues hitherto unknown. Some did not even bother to spell out their theoretical foundations, nor to substantiate their claims to better results.

Under these conditions it becomes mandatory to offer a thumbnail sketch and clarification of the basic concepts of whatever approach one deals with, in this case the Rogerian, which is, incidentally, the most empirically researched among the multitude now existant and the first to be exclusively and thoroughly novel, both in its theory[1] and its strikingly revolutionary practice. Also, Rogerian therapy was the first to be typically North American in the sense of reflecting the ideals of the North American way of life: democracy, autonomy, and private enterprise.

What's in a Name

Most urgently in need of clarification is the term "nondirective." While this label was long ago discarded by Carl R. Rogers and his fellow workers, it remains stubbornly anchored in the memory of layman and professional alike. This first name was given, somewhat hesitantly, when Rogers's work was still in the early stages of its emergence as a distinctly new concept. A concept characterized by its bold departures from the only system then in existence and at that time regarded as the only one conceivable: psychoanalysis. The revolutionary character of this novel approach was soon recognized, and the demand for dissemination and publication became pressing. A title was needed. Naturally, the title was chosen to reflect the most characteristic feature of the subject. From the point of view of the observer, that feature obviously consisted of the absence of directions, either implicit under the guise of questions or comments or explicit in the form of outright exploration, guidance, and advice. Not surprisingly, the label "nondirective" was proposed, and it was accepted with some hesitation. Rogers himself was not yet quite sure just what was the crucial factor in the approach he was still in the process of developing.

However, it did not take long before he realized that the mere absence of directions could not account for the results that seemed to flow from his work. In the process of his ongoing research, he and his associates were faced with a puzzling fact that led to a critically significant insight. In studying their recorded interviews they found that whenever his coworkers tried their hand at this approach, faithfully imitating Rogers in avoiding all questions, interpretations, or guidance, no results seemed forthcoming. Clients declared themselves dissatisfied, felt bored, and promptly terminated the interviews. During the regular discussion sessions that Rogers entertained with his fellow clinical psychologists at Ohio State University, these puzzling occurrences were carefully scrutinized. Thus it was discovered that Rogers held significantly different attitudes and beliefs about clients than did those who had unsuccessfully tried his style of interaction. It became apparent that what others regarded as a _technique_ was to Rogers a _belief_. It was a firm belief in people's capacity to perform the essentials of the job by themselves, if given a fair chance, as in a propitious human relationship.

This belief was not just a personal bent; it was the product of countless earlier observations. Among these was that his clients tended to delay dealing with their problems, in their own terms rather than in the assumedly more realistic terms of the expert. Also, they seemed able to make judgments and draw conclusions better suited to their _felt_ needs than the judgements and conclusions of the therapist, which were probably more accurate but somehow foreign to their way of perceiving. This reminded him of another astounding observation he had made in the early days of his work (conducted then in terms of his training[2]), namely that the more accurate his interpretations, the stronger the clients' resistance or opposition. Pondering all this, he began to rely more and more upon the client's initiatives, without reinforcing in either direction, but also without judging or correcting. Gradually he found himself adopting an increasingly other-centered, empathic attitude. Thus, "client-centered" came to replace "nondirective" as a more intrinsically suitable designation for his work.

However, just as the old label "nondirective"

was a misnomer, so also the new designation "client-centered" failed to do justice to the essence of Rogers's thinking. Indeed, when used in an absurdly external sense, "client-centered" could be taken to mean something that is part of the very structure of any therapy, since the client is by definition the center of the process, insofar as he or she is its subject and assumed beneficiary. However, as will appear from the following explanations, the operational (as distinct from the nominal) significance of the term is radically different, indeed, revolutionarily so. No single benchmark sort of a word can reveal the essence of as complex a notion as psychotherapy. Even "psychoanalysis," now a household word, was initially an obscure notion, hermetically closed to the layman. It stirred curiosity as a nearly occult process bringing to light deeply hidden and troublesome material, to be "exorcised" by the analyst, instead of being regarded as a type of treatment.

Something of the same fate, but in reverse, awaited Rogers's labels. While the word "psychoanalysis" was initially so obscure as to awe the outsider, so the terms "nondirective" and "client-centered" were considered so self-explanatory, so transparent, as to dispense the newcomer from any serious effort at exploring their meaning. Similarly, their application in practice seemed too simple to require specific training. Little did the would-be practitioner understand how deceptive that simplicity was, and how critical the creation of conducive conditions would be to an awakening of dormant capacities. To my view, it seems likely that significant change must take place within each practitioner, before that practitioner can function in an authentically empathic manner, which is a main condition for the practice of this approach.

In hindsight, it is clear that the most appropriate label for a body of thought and manner of interacting such as devised by Rogers would have been humanistic--expressive of the value of the human being, of the respect due that persons's aspiration toward autonomy, tendencies toward existential competence, and nearly limitless potential. But the term humanistic had not yet penetrated the hard-core mechanistic-deterministic philosophy of psychology at the time the Rogers approach (May et al., 1958) appeared on the scene.

BASIC CONCEPTS

The basic concepts of Rogerian theory and practice can coherently be formulated in two propositions.

1. The human being has the capacity, potential if not actual, and the tendency, to his or her own self and problems to the extent necessary to take constructive action.
2. This capacity becomes actualized in a relationship that is free from threat to the self; that is, a relationship characterized by empathic understanding, unconditional regard; and authenticity.

These are not just "words, words, words." They are well considered statements, pared to the bare bones. Every single word counts. Take away one or two and the whole loses its validity. Because these terms are so pregnant with meaning, it is important, and, even interesting, to get acquainted with them one by one.

Proposition 1

<u>"The human being . . ."</u>

This concept is taken in its most encompassing sense, referring not only to the intelligent, the educated, or the privileged but to the average human being, functioning with a working measure of awareness and ability to communicate.

<u>"has the capacity, potential if not actual . . ."</u>

Often underrated but of central importance here is the qualifier "potential," necessary to lend credibility to the affirmation of human capacity, the key concept of this approach.

Unfortunately, most individuals live and perform considerably below their potential. This happens not for lack of desire to enhance themselves, to make the most of their existence, but for lack of the awareness and self-confidence they need to strike out at available opportunities and test themselves at new learning, new tasks. Many live as if their present condition were their destiny. Their capacities are dormant for lack of conditions favorable to their development. Or they are blocked by rules and customs they consider unchangeable.

Therefore their underlying potential increasingly resists actualization and gradually deteriorates, unless it becomes vivified and energized by some stirring event, random or planned.

The most basic feature of organisms is their tendency toward orthogenic growth according to a built-in blueprint. In the human organism this tendency, though equally strong, but beyond the strictly physical, is not guided by an intrinsic model. Its most basic features are its plasticity, its versatility, and its protean nature. Indeed, the actualization of this potential may express itself in almost any shape, behavior, or attitude called out by environmental determinants. At the same time, it is always aiming at its own enhancement as perceived at any point in time.

<u>"and the tendency . . ."</u>

"The tendency": This clause expresses what is perhaps the most dynamic ingredient in the process of converting potentiality into actuality. In a therapeutic context, this tendency is the yeast in the loaf, the springboard which accounts for the possibility of genuine and enduring change. Without life's built-in tendency to move forward and upward, it is doubtful much would be accomplished even under the best of conditions.

Curiously, the power of this vital force is often overlooked in discussions on the subject. It is an idea that, even now, runs counter to a deeply rooted cultural stereotype according to which, in matters of treatment, positive change can come about only through external, expert action. The idea that constructive change can come about <u>through the release of forces from within</u> is still too novel to dispel the effect of lingering mechanistic thinking.

Often forgotten or underestimated is the fact that organisms are bundles of tendencies without which most learning would either be impossible or not lasting. Psychologists' emphasis upon the universal capacity of organisms for adaptation and learning is well known and abundantly supported both experimentally and empirically. However, not all of these capacities are boosted by tendencies. Thus, one of the duckling's earliest behaviors is to swim if water is available. Such behavior is backed by tendency. Not so that of the young chick. It will not wet its toes except from necessity to drink. To train it to engage in swimming freely might be possible but would not be lasting.

Similarly, 60 years ago experiments with human subjects demonstrated (Stratton, 1929) that they are able to manage effectively in surroundings reversed in a radically upside down direction, by the use of spectacles designed to make this tour de force possible. But none of these subjects showed any inclination to adopt this capacity as part of ordinary living. More currently, in most, if not all universities, one of the requirements for a doctoral degree is a dissertation based upon research in either laboratory or library. Practically all the candidates succeed in completing this (frequently detested) requirement. But follow-ups (Shakow, 1978) show that the percentage of those who choose to engage freely in further research is soberingly slim.

The ability to learn a skill is one thing. To adopt it as a way of life, quite another. In therapy, this ability to incorporate change is the sine qua non of lasting change. If the change were not supported by the tendency toward self-enhancement, even the best efforts to bring it about would be futile.

"to understand his or her own self and problems . . ."

This part of the proposition is the one most readily attacked by the outsider as unrealistic and unworthy of further attention. Actually, need it really be made plain that the understanding meant here is nothing like the academic, technical understanding of the professional? It is not diagnostic or psychodynamic in any formal sense. Indeed, it is inconceivable that the layman could diagnose himself with the precision and accuracy of the specialist, that is, with the precision and accuracy of his formulation. However, what matters here is not the formulation but the understanding, the actual, living understanding, perhaps unformulated but existential, capable of serving as a basis for real change.

"to the extent necessary to take constructive action."

The moderation of this clause is likely to calm the antagonism aroused by the preceding one, the earlier affirmation of the client's capacity to understand himself, or herself, from which it should perhaps not be separated. Indeed, it does not say that human beings have the capacity to cure or restore themselves to full functioning, or to make their lives problem proof. That would rudely fly in the face of common sense. What it does say is that, under specific conditions such as those that will be described here, constructive action is well-nigh bound to occur, however modest that action may be at the start. At a minimum it might consist of a mere good feeling, gained sometimes from the first contact, leading to a continuation of the often skeptically started enterprise. A growing feeling of self-respect and competence tends to develop. In due course this feeling becomes rewarding enough to motivate the client toward tackling life anew, this time with more insight and renewed confidence.

A characteristic difference between self-directed and other-directed therapy usually lies in the scope of the change the client and practitioner set as their goal. The professional typically aims at the personality as a whole, at the complex system of needs and inclinations that constitute the basic self. The professional's ideal is to perform a thorough job designed to equip the client with a blueprint of his or her self-structure, its tendencies and liabilities. A blueprint that may enable the holder to meet constructively whatever vicissitudes life may hold in store.

The client, on the other hand, may not be ready for as deeply probing a job. The concern of the client tends to lie with the problems at hand: with the unhappiness of the moment, as the client perceives it, however incomplete or mistaken his or her views may be at the time. The client will grow who feels that the therapist takes him or her seriously, that the therapist understands and accepts his or her views; that the therapist refrains from challenging them, from expressing doubts or judgments. Instead, if the therapist consistently lends an intense and sustaining attention, voices only brief indications as to how deeply he or she understands, the client may go a long way. It should be emphasized again and again: The therapist should be consistently careful to indicate that his or her acceptance and understanding shows concern for the client's <u>feelings</u> and <u>perceptions</u>, not necessarily the <u>facts</u> as reported.

At the start, the self-propelled process consists of a random groping, leading to scattered glimpses of insight into the problem and the self. These glimpses gradually coalesce and turn into a sort of loose structure-in-motion. Parts of that nebulous structure tend to consolidate, others to fade away, while others again emerge filling the gaps.

The client gains a dawning feeling that things are beginning to fall into place. This random process of exploration, evaluation, and modification acquires increasing direction and moves toward the discovery of that cluster of needs and values that constitutes the real, operational self. In light of that discovery, the target problem, that brought the client to the therapist, begins to be seen in a different light in which it seems amenable to solution. In the successful case this ability to test, check, and scrutinize the self far outlasts the period of therapeutic contacts. It tends to become part of the client's makeup and to operate in an informal, as it were organic, way. A fascinating process to behold.

Proposition 2:

The above presented high-minded and generous concepts would have little to stand on in practice without their complementary part: the necessary and sufficient conditions. Again we will engage in a one-by-one commentary on these key terms. Actually, much about these has already been presented in the analysis of Proposition 1, since being that they are inseparable twins.

It may be helpful first to repeat the proposition in its entirety: This capacity becomes actualized in <u>a relationship</u> that is <u>free from threat to the self</u>; that is, a relationship characterized by <u>empathic understanding, unconditional regard, and authenticity</u>.

The first requirement, then, is

<u>"relationship . . ."</u>

Whenever two or more people are freely engaged in some enterprise there is a relationship. Good, bad, or somewhere in between. For obvious reasons, we will limit ourselves to the good kind of relationships. Their qualitative diversity is endless, depending on the kinds of pursuits and feelings involved. Despite all their diversity, one can discern certain fundamental features common to all. They are person-to-person relationships, genuine and egalitarian. The parties are mindful of the fact that each has a fund of experience, and the capacity and right to think and to speak in his or her own rights. Also that each has vulnerability, which may not show but which has to be kept in mind.

In the complex fabric of human interaction, the quality of the relationship is often regarded as a mere frill, something imponderable with little bearing on the substance of the issues, a bonus. Actually, far from being trivial, the relationship is of central importance to many enterprises. In many cases it is the backbone of their viability. The creation of such a relationship is the key task of the therapist. It should be:

"free from threat to the self . . ."

Threat to the self consists in anything which the individual perceives as inconsistent with the image of himself or herself. Anything that differs or tends to diminish that image threatens and leads to defensiveness. Such inconsistencies are perceived as outright wrong, unjust, offensive, painful. Hence the individual tends to resist, resent, or reject them as personal attacks and ceases to disclose himself or herself.

In this connection let us present a graphic example: Take a client who is a mother and displays an all-absorbing, totally self-sacrificing love and care for her child, with whom, incidentally, nothing seems wrong, and a therapist who has come to know this mother as deeply neurotic. Suppose the therapist believes in helping this client by tactfully confronting her with reality. He attempts to open her eyes by explaining (on the basis of undeniable evidence) that her self-sacrificing way of life is actually a way of using her child as a front to hide some secret design, to monopolize the child's affection, elicit jealousy, take revenge or some other wretched thing of the kind. This well meaning therapist is likely to see a sweet and tender-minded person turn into a menacing mountain cat: someone has seen through her most clever schemes! She feels powerless, angry, resentful, destroyed. Attempts to resume contact are out of the question.

Conversely, if the therapist fully enters the frame of reference of this client, leaving aside his or her own sense of reality, rationality, and common sense, that is, his or her own frame of reference, for the purpose of removing all threat to the client, that therapist is likely to recognize signs of the client's urge to be relieved of the burden of her duplicity. Feeling safe, she is apt to gradually reveal the schemes she is "compelled" to set up and to "justify"; she begins to doubt their effectiveness, to evaluate their emotional cost, to foresee that they may ultimately boomerang. Finally she is likely to drop them, with understandable reluctance but firm resolve, ultimately perhaps with eagerness. A sense of legitimate pride in her accomplishments is reward enough to lead toward adopting the relieving habit of being open with herself. Congratulations on the part of the therapist are not needed; they would only alter the sense of existential reward. She knows that the therapist realizes, beyond words.

"empathic understanding . . ."

Complete freedom from threat can be achieved only via empathic understanding. No amount of reassurance as to the safety of the situation and the secrecy of the communication can create the feeling of security required to induce the client to bare the smallish, ungenuine, tricky, or wicked features of the self. The condemning codes of society and morality sometimes have too strong a hold upon the individual to permit him or her to acknowledge, even to a single outsider, the existence of these socially condemned features within the otherwise decent self. How then can this material come to the surface? This can happen only in conditions of empathic understanding, the key to safety from threat to the self.

An example from everyday life may be helpful here. Many of us have had the opportunity to observe, and some the privilege of interacting with, that rare human specimen, a remarkably unaggressive, mild, and quiet person with whom it feels good to have an encounter. Such persons are not necessarily highly educated, informed, or trained, but they have a particular make-up with a subdued appeal all its own. They are able to listen in an engaging and affable manner without manifesting any need to interrupt with questions or comments, favorable or unfavorable, or to bring up anything that might stem the flow of the speaker's outpouring. Such persons are somehow good company, often sought after to share particular experiences or private revelations. They are eminently empathic by nature.

Quite different is the typical model of everyday interaction. Parties take turns listening and replying; they agree/disagree, persuade/approve, deplore/congratulate, point out where one is right/the other wrong, and the whole gamut; all of this comes strictly from their own frames of reference, from their views of what is real, good, or true. Active participation is about equal. Parties who approve or agree at every turn are soon considered boring. Especially shunned are those who always seem to know better. Obviously this type of interaction is the direct opposite of empathic understanding.

Unless a genuine capacity for empathy is part of one's makeup, it is doubtful one would practice it for any length of time for the fun of it. To be able and willing to adopt it as a therapeutic style of interaction requires a keen insight into the dynamics of this unimpressive, subdued, yet powerful kind of encounter, conducted entirely within the frame of reference of only one party. Such interaction makes for a feeling of safety unmatched by any other. Neither the content nor the accuracy of the communication is in danger of being questioned, criticized, or tested.

The client begins to feel relieved from the tension of his or her usually guarded and defensive attitude and becomes able to "let go." After the experience of such free flowing self-expression, the client also tends to become capable of reviewing and modifying some of his or her unchecked, uncontrolled utterances.

At this point a truly remarkable thing occurs: <u>When the listener refrains from performing the role of the critic, the speaker tends to assume that role</u> (Rogers, 1951). Wanting to keep or restore his or her own self-respect as a fairly reasonable person, the client begins to realize that here and there, he or she has exaggerated or otherwise distorted certain things. The client starts rounding off some of the sharpened edges of his or her reports, makes some concessions, and grants some points to whatever or whomever is the subject of the ire, hurt, and upset. The client's better self tends to move to the surface, and he or she becomes able to resume "business as usual," often more constructively and at less emotional cost than ever before.

Need it be pointed out that all this does not occur overnight? It is a process, initially with uncertain direction, set in motion by the facilitating attitude of the one who shares, as it were, the relieving flood of pent-up emotion. From a rambling start it grows into a more or less rationally checked, goal-directed process that continues in between meetings in an increasingly self-propelled, problem-solving direction.

The reader may feel such humble results are out of proportion with the efforts of the parties, at least with those of the therapist who has to create the rather taxing conditions required to obtain results via this model of interaction. There is a point to this. Whether or not one chooses to carry the burden that falls on the therapist in this method is a matter of values and philosophy of life. The therapist who places high value on helping the client to become a person (Rogers, 1951), not simply an adjusted or successful member of his or her culture, will not be deterred by the effort to be expended. Furthermore, awareness of the fact that one is working in the evolutionary direction of human relations (toward the "Person-to-Person" and away from the "Agent-to-Object" model, Buber, 1937) is generally felt as sufficiently compensating for the serious humanist.

Some readers may be disappointed to find that this approach yields nothing of the kind of Luminous Transformation, Rebirth, or Liberation touted by what Michael Konner (Kinget, 1975) calls the "late-night TV psycho-babble." Indeed, there is nothing flashy about this approach, for it refers to the phenomenon of growth, not remodeling, and growth is not visible to the naked eye. Also, much essential growth occurs underground. But when growth slowly emerges into bud and blossom, it fills us with surprise and, in most cases, with delight.

"unconditional regard . . ."

The term "regard" refers to a blend of respect, concern, and trust, not simply to warmth and civility, which must be taken for granted in delicate situations of this kind. Regard, then, is indispensable for the activation of potentiality. Hence it is crucial that the concept be clearly understood.

Unfortunately, two of its ingredients are particularly apt to cause controversy, even near outrage. The newcomer to this way of thinking tends to feel indignant, to scoff at the idea of placing unconditional trust and respect in the kind of individual one is apt to meet in therapeutic practice. "Who would or could genuinely respect a child molester, a sadist, an arsonist?", "Who could trust an embezzler, a confirmed cheater or perjurer?", it is argued. Indeed, who could? Who would?

The answer is that the object of the regard here referred to is not the individual insofar as that individual is a criminal, an exploiter, or a cheater. It is addressed to that part of the potential self that is not actualized, that can be reached only via close acquaintance with the client's perceptual world as such. This in turn can take place only if the client feels that he or she is treated with genuine regard, encompassing all of himself or herself, the bad, but also the good.

This trust and respect can be genuine only when they flow from a deep belief in the unlimited potential, in those parts that are not realized but contain forces capable of bringing the client to the point of wanting to change, to cease being what he or she has been so far and to elicit the desire for a more humanly rewarding way of life. A potential that perhaps did not have a chance at actualization under the conditions of the social, moral, and material world in which the individual developed.[3] If the client feels that the therapist takes him or her seriously; genuinely accepts his or her reports; manifests the fullest attention and consistent respect; avoids all interruption; makes all comments, favorable or otherwise, giving only brief indications as to how deeply he or she understands, then the client will open up. The client's views will tend to become amenable to redefinition. This redefinition occurs, again, largely in his or her own terms, but this time the terms are more accurate, more apt to come closer to the reality of things, more amenable to constructive change.

Again, in all this, it is absolutely crucial that the therapist be careful not to mislead the client into believing that the understanding and acceptance offered concern not the <u>facts</u> of the reports but the genuineness of the reports as he or she <u>perceives</u> them.

<u>"authenticity."</u>

To the necessity for authenticity, mentioned repeatedly throughout these pages, little remains to be added. From the section dealing with Rogers's early work, when his coworkers regarded his nondirectiveness as a technique instead of a philosophy-in-action, down to these last pages, reminders have been dropped about the importance of this attitude. Furthermore, in the word "authentic," used here in its common meaning of genuine, sincere, free from make-believe, there is little danger of misunderstanding.

One thing, however, should be made clear. The

authenticity here insisted upon does not refer to the therapist as a private person; in private life the therapist need not be more genuine, truthful, straightforward, or sincere than his or her colleagues. It refers solely to his or her willingness and ability to forget values, so as to be free to enter the client's frame of reference and able to genuinely practice the empathy and positive regard here required. Of course, the more genuine the person is by nature, the easier it will be to satisfy this requirement. Those not so inclined, are likely to change their attitudes once they have the opportunity to observe directly the dynamics of genuine empathy.

One question remains; it concerns the possibility for the therapist to be authentic while at the same time remaining himself or herself, with his or her own personal views and values. The question is a realistic one. The answer can only partially be put into words. Therapeutic authenticity requires that the therapist step deliberately outside his or her own frame of reference, leaving it behind in order to immerse himself or herself as fully as possible into the frame of reference of another, the client, though only for the duration of the interaction. But this only moves the question one step further.

What is empathic understanding? In other words; what is "genuinely entering into another's frame of reference." It is not a skill that can be picked up at will, like baseball or cards. Actually, it seems more and more likely that a certain self change, a certain growth has to take place within the therapist. Such takes time. What in the meantime?

For those who do not have the opportunity of training with a first-class therapist of this persuasion, as I was privileged to have with Rogers himself, I might offer the following thought.

I have often observed here, as in other domains, (and so perhaps have you) that the presence of an intense desire, an eagerness to acquire a certain quality or skill may obtain results that gradually become comparable to the established possession of that skill. To coin a phrase; practice makes perfect.[4]

A FINAL POINT

The goal of virtually all therapies is to solve the problem, to cure or change the client. Like most enterprises, the process of psychotherapy is seen as a process of roughly estimated duration with a distinct beginning and end. The beginning is set by the client if the client initiates the action, that is, is not referred by another, such as a physician, relative, or friend. As a rule the end is set by the therapist on the basis of the therapist's perceptions and experience, his or her feeling of "closure."

Quite different is Rogers's concept of the undertaking, especially with respect to the length of therapy and "termination" of the process. In his own felicitously chosen words, "psychotherapy is a journey, not a destination" (Rogers, 1951). For the process does not, should not, end when the interviews cease. Ideally it is a lifetime process. Life is a problem-solving task from beginning to end; therefore Rogers's concept of the therapeutic goal is essentially to offer the client an opportunity to acquire self-helping capacity and problem-solving attitudes for lifetime use.

NOTES

1. "Every new theoretical contribution in the field of psychotherapy which has had the originality and germinating power to lead to the developing of a new school has come from continental Europe with only two exceptions--and, of these, one was grandsired by a European-born psychiatrist." (May et al., 1959, p. 9). The other was Carl R. Rogers, the only psychologist to conceptualize an entirely novel, purely North American approach--egalitarian, democratic, and humanistic.

2. Rogers himself had been trained in the psychoanalytic tradition, there being no other approach at the time. His mentors were notable in New York, analysts for whom he kept a lifelong respect, despite their deep variances on the subject of their professional endeavors.

3. This is not to support a belief in the hard kind of determinism according to which the individual is the exclusive product of social forces and, of course, heredity. It is only to remind the reader of the staggering influence these determinants exert upon that potential. Indeed, these influences are the inherently protean, ever incipient forces from within, often beleaguered, opposed, or baited by the social-cultural forces that inevitably constitute their environment.

4. Those who want to learn more about the "how to" of this approach I might refer to a work I published with Rogers in several languages, the second volume of which deals mainly with the "how to" of this approach, reported in the bibliography (Rogers and Kinget, 1959; 1970).

REFERENCES

Buber, M. 1937. I and Thou. Edinburgh: Clark.

Herrink, R. 1980. Psychotherapy Handbook: The E-Z Guide to More Than 250 Psychotherapies. New York: New American Library.

Kinget, G. M. 1962. Psychotherapie et Relations Humaines. Vol. 2. Paris and Louvain: Nauwelaerts. (1965; 2nd ed.)

Kinget, G. M. 1967. Psicoterapia y Relaciones Humanas. Vol. 2. (Translation.) Orense, Spain: Ediciones Alfaguara.

Kinget, G. M. 1975. On Being Human. San Francisco: Harcourt Brace Jovanovich.

Konner, M. 1982. The Tangled Wing. New York: Holt, Rinehart, Winston.

May, R., E. Angel, and H. Ellenberger, Eds. Existence. New York: Basic Books.

Rogers, C. R. 1951. Client-Centered Therapy. Boston: Houghton Mifflin.

Rogers, C. R. 1961. On Becoming A Person. Boston: Houghton Mifflin.

Rogers, C. R. and Kinget, G. M. 1959. Psychotherapie en Menselijke Verhoudingen. Utrecht, Netherlands: Uitgeverij Het Spectrum. (1974; paperback ed.)

Rogers, C. R. and Kinget, G. M. 1970. Psicoterapia e Relazioni Umane. (Translation.) Torino, Italy: Boringhieri.

Shakow, D. 1978. "Clinical Psychology Seen Some 50 Years Later." American Psychologist, 33; no. 2 (February): 148-58.

Stratton, G. M. 1929. "Vision Without Inversion of the Retinal Image." In E. G. Boring. History of Experimental Psychology. 2nd ed. New York and London: Century, p. 689.

7

The Nature of Psychopathology

Mark H. Bickhard

In this chapter I wish to address the question of the nature of psychopathology. It might naturally be felt that we already know a great deal about psychopathology, and thus that such a chapter would be primarily a review and discussion of the literature. I will argue, however, that the most fundamental form of the question concerning the nature of psychopathology is rarely posed in the literature, that it is prevented from being posed by presuppositions inherent in standard theoretical approaches, and that, on those rare occasions when it has been addressed, it has received inadequate answers. Therefore the chapter will have more of the character of a conceptual explication and theoretical exegesis than it will of a review of the literature. The chapter is structural in two general parts: (1) a brief summary of standard approaches and their inadequacies; and (2) an explication and explanation of psychopathology as a manifestation of certain properties of experiential processes.

STANDARD APPROACHES

Typologies and Models

Discussions of psychopathology commonly consist of typologies of presumed <u>forms</u> of psychopathology. The focus is on descriptive and diagnostic criteria and on the usefulness of the resultant categories for research, bureaucratic record keeping, treatment planning, and so on. Such criterial considerations may be approached within the still current (within psychology) myth of operational definitionalism (Bickhard, et al., 1985; Suppe, 1973; 1977), in which case the primary concerns will be with various forms of psychometric validity, with essentially no attention to the issues of the underlying ontology the basic nature, of the presumed categories. Alternatively, the typology of psychopathology may be generated within the framework of a personality theory, which personality theory may then implicitly or explicitly provide an underlying ontology for the categories.

What is common to the two typological approaches is that the categories of psychopathology are proposed as types of potential _dysfunctionality_, with no further attention given to the nature of those dysfunctionalities and, in particular, no attention given to the question of what it is that makes those dysfunctionalities _pathological_. The issue that I wish to raise here is not that the forms of psychopathology commonly described are not in fact pathological (that point might in fact be argued for some of the diagnostic categories, but that is not my current concern), but rather that their pathological nature is taken for granted (it is "obvious" from the descriptions that "this" constitutes a pathology) and that the fundamental nature of psychopathology is thus never examined and, correspondingly, never understood. In general, what _is_ obvious about such categories is that they seem in varying degrees and in varying ways dysfunctional and that, since psychopathology per se is not examined, dysfunctionality and psychopathology are implicitly equated. As will be argued, this is deeply false.

Psychopathology as Rigidity

The equating of psychopathology and dysfunctionality is in effect an equating of psychopathology with ignorance and error. Ignorance and error are problems that inevitably confront everyone. They are unavoidable, and they inherently, by definition, produce dysfunctionality or reduced functionality. To equate psychopathology and dysfunctionality is to render all people inevitably pathological simply by virtue of their finiteness (finiteness makes ignorance and error), thus dysfunctionality, under this "analysis," into an existential certainty. This is a nugatory explication of psychopathology (it does not do the work of differentiating anything from anything, since it applies to everyone) and is clearly not what anyone intends, but it is what the simple-minded equating of psychopathology and dysfunctionality entails.

A more careful approach to psychopathology might attempt to explicate it as a certain kind (or kinds) of dysfunctionality, leaving the dysfunctionalities of simple ignorance and error aside. This approach, however, raises exactly the question of what psychopathology is, other than, or in addition to, dysfunctionality. What is the differentiating characteristic? One superficially immediate answer would be that psychopathological dysfunctionality is more serious than simple ignorance or error. Unfortunately, however, "simple" ignorance or error can be fatal, and some neuroses may be merely restricting or discomforting. A distiction based on "seriousness of consequences" does not fare well. I will argue, in fact, that psychopathology is not a kind of dysfunctionality at all and, correspondingly, that its relationship to dysfunctionality is more complex than that of genus to species.

In particular, I would suggest that a valid explication of the notion of psychopathology is that psychopathology is constituted as <u>rigidity</u>. It is not being ignorant nor being in error that constitutes psychopathology; it is the persistence of such ignorance and error in the face of sometimes massive and repetitive dysfunctionality, and in spite of the potentially desperate efforts of intelligent, motivated, and creative individuals to change. The paradigmatic form of psychopathology is the individual who even understands the pattern of his or her dysfunctionality, but whose every attempt to change that pattern manages to perpetuate it. Ignorance and error that is correctable by simple feedback or information is not pathological (Bickhard and Ford, 1979). Psychopathology is the rigidity of some way of being in the world. (This notion of rigidity is broader than the important explication of "rigid character" in Shapiro, 1981.)

It should be noted that the explication of psychopathology as rigidity shifts the focus of the concept from a relational consideration to an intrinsic consideration. Dysfunctionality is inherently a relational concept: one is dysfunctional only in or with respect to particular environments or situations. Rigidity is an inherent property of a person's way of being: the potentiality for, the openness to, change is present or absent independently of what happens to be the current situation or the current feedback that an individual is receiving. It would be possible within this explication for someone to instantiate an extremely rigid, thus pathological, way of being that happens to be in an environment in which that way of being is appropriate and adaptive, or functional. It would also be possible for someone to manifest a strong dysfunctionality by various external criteria, but for whom that way of being was a full and open choice based on nonintrinsically rigid values. This explication, in other words, splits the notion of psychopathology from that of social deviance and thus avoids the dangers of abuse, as well as relativism, inherent in that mode. In practice most of the instances of psychopathology that one encounters will also be instances of dysfunctionality, but that is not an inherent constraint in this explication.

Structural Models of Psychopathology

The association of rigidity with psychopathology has certainly been noted before, and it has a feel of obviousness once pointed out, but it is rarely given the emphasis, the explicatory essentialness, that I am proposing for it. Within the majority of current approaches to the nature of the person there are good reasons for this: the person is conceived of as being essentially structural in nature, and structures are intrinsically rigid. Rigidity is part of the meaning of what it is to be a structure, thus rigidity needs no independent explanation or explanatory model. If, for example, a certain form of psychopathology is presumed to be constituted as a particular structure of introjected object fragments and corresponding fragments of the self, then the persistence, the rigidity, of that structure needs no independent explanation: such a structure _is_ the person, and structures are intrinsically rigid.

The fundamental question from such a perspective, in fact, is not the question of rigidity; it is the problem of change: if a person is intrinsically structural, thus intrinsically rigid, then how does change (to a new, presumably less dysfunctional structure) ever occur (Gendlin, 1970)? Note that if persons are intrinsically structural, then they are intrinsically rigid, and psychopathology _must_ be equated with certain forms of dysfunctionality, since the property of (structural) rigidity, per se, is common to everyone. The goal of therapy in such a perspective is to change a more dysfunctional structure into a less dysfunctional structure, but if the person is ontologically structural, then there is no intrinsic process by which that change can occur. At best, the process by which an individual can and does expand his or her way of living, by which an individual can overcome rigid dysfunctions, remains utterly mysterious, with correspondingly little or no guidance to the therapist in how to nurture and encourage that process. At worst, there is no way for that structure, that person, to change itself--there is no process in the model. Any change must be the result of an external intervention from the beneficent therapist. Structural models allow at most a state change model: If such and such is the current state, then creating XYZ conditions will yield a change from that (structural) state to this other (structural) state. (Note that this is the basic logical form of "treatment strategies.") Structural models can define change, as a change in structure, and they can conceivably give recipes for externally induced medical-model interventions, but they cannot explain, cannot aid, self change. Without a process model of the nature of the person, they cannot accommodate the phenomena of personal growth, and therefore cannot guide the therapist with respect to it.

However, with a process model of the nature of the person, (with a fundamental conception of persons as being in process and in development, as being continually and intrinsically growing and developing from at least birth onward), the basic question shifts from one of how could change possibly occur to one of how could rigidity possibly occur. Rigidity is intrinsic to the nature of the person within a structural perspective, and thus needs no independent explanation, but (the potentiality for) change is intrinsic to the person within a process perspective, and thus rigidity does need an explanation. Furthermore, if the ontology of person is fundamentally one of a self-organizing open system, the rigidity not only needs explanation, it is intrinsically a blockage of, a violation of, that ontology--it is intrinsically pathological. Within a structural view, therapy consists of the induction of change; within a process view, therapy consists of the freeing from rigidity.

Process versus Structural Models

Once the problem of rigidity is recognized as a distinct issue in its own right, it becomes a powerful question to bring to bear on proffered models of personality and psychopathology. With respect to a purported explication of psychopathology, the basic question is: "How and why does the purported psychopathological structure or pattern stay that way?" That is, "How and why is it rigid?". Any model that explicitly or implicitly responds to such a question by referring to the structural character of the "disorder" is engaged in question begging. Structures are intrinsically rigid, so a question of how and why such and such a condition remains rigid is in effect a question concerning the justification for modeling it in a structural form in the first place. Structures simply presuppose rigidity they do not explicate nor explain it. So to answer that a condition is rigid because it is structural is in effect to answer that it is rigid because it is rigid--the basic question has not been addressed.

Structural models may sound as if they at least address the general issue of pathological rigidity, but most often they simply provide some version of the nature of dysfunctionality, with the property of rigidity implicit in the structural character of the model. Psychopathology as the filtering of information, from the environment or from the purported "unconscious," provides a common category of examples. Something akin to such filtering certainly does seem to occur, at least in some cases, but the fundamental modeling question is how such a filtering process could maintain itself, how it could persist, how it could be rigid. There is no answer except the implicit allusion to the structural nature of the model. For this type of model there is even a deep logical problem concerning the fact that any meaningful filtering must involve knowledge of what something is, in order to know whether or not to filter it, but such knowledge is precisely what the filtering was presumed to be preventing. If the person, per se, is presumed to be doing the filtering, then we have the paradox of someone continuing to be successful in lying to himself or herself. If a separate homunculus, that is, a censor, is invented to "solve" this problem (the censor "knows" and can filter therapies, but the person is thereby prevented from knowing), then we are already in the realm of structural models. The censoring agent is somehow structurally different from the person agent, and in any case, the logical problem simply recurs in the form of a metafiltering, a metacensoring, of the activities of the censor (resistance). The censor may be filtering from the person, but what prevents the person from discovering, from learning about, the activities of the censor? What makes such filtering rigid? What filters the filtering? The problem simply iterates and initiates an infinite regress. Whatever role informational filtering may or may not have in psychopathology, it cannot constitute the fundamental ground of psychopathology because it cannot in itself explain the core phenomenon of rigidity. It cannot explain why people don't self-organize, learn, their way out of such filtering as a result of the postulated dysfunctionalities of that filtering.

Another common attempt at explicating psychopathology does have a process character, but it also does not ultimately succeed in solving the basic problem of rigidity. This is the attempted explication of psychopathology in terms of self-fulfilling prophecy (e.g., Wachtel, 1973). The basic idea is that an individual acts in the world in accordance with certain generically incorrect or incomplete expectations and assumptions concerning himself or herself or the world, and that those actions induce reactions from other people that fulfill those expectations and confirm those assumptions. Again, this certainly occurs, but the phenomenon is never perfect; there are variations in people's reactions; there are exceptions to the expectations; and the question remains of why and how the individual doesn't differentiate the underlying expectations and assumptions in accordance with such feedback. Why doesn't the individual learn when those assumptions are likely to be appropriate and when not? Why doesn't he or she learn the way right out of the dysfunctionality? Why is the self-fulfilling cycle itself rigid? There is no answer within a structuralist framework.

A PROCESS MODEL OF PSYCHOPATHOLOGICAL RIGIDITY

The first step in the development of a process model of psychopathology has already been taken: the explication of psychopathology as rigidity. The next is to explain how such rigidity could occur, and that will be addressed in two parts: first, a functional account of how rigidity is possible and, second, a process account of how such a functional property could be instantiated. There, then, follows a discussion of some additional ontological and functional characteristics of psychopathology as it is generally found in the individual.

Rigidity as Autoprotectiveness

The fundamental nature of the problem of rigidity is to explain how some particular way of being maintains itself, how it manages not to process change. If the answer is in terms of some _other_ process that protects the given process from change, then the question simply reverts to that second process--what keeps it rigid? Such derivative rigidity does certainly occur (in fact, such _derivatively_ rigid distortions of functioning constitute most _presented_ pathology), but foundational rigidity cannot be explained in such a form on pain of infinite regress. Somehow, the rigidity of a foundationally pathological way of being in the world must be explicable in terms of that way of being itself. Somehow the way of being must intrinsically prevent its own change, must be _autoprotective_.

The issue here is not that the pathological way of being is unchangeable, but rather that it is deeply impeded from changing itself. For it to be unchangeable would be for it to be rigidly structural in the worst sense, and by definition no therapeutic intervention would be possible. For it to be unable to change itself entails that whatever _would_ change it is prevented by it. A pathological way of being must prevent, must forbid, precisely those forms of self-examination, problem solving, or whatever would be required to change that way of being. It must protect itself against the discovery of its implicit error or limitation. A psychopathological way of being is so by virtue of being rigid, and it is rigid by virtue of being autoprotective.

Characteristics of Autoprotective Processes

Autoprotectiveness, then, is a functional explication of rigidity, and thus of psychopathology, but in itself that does not explain how autoprotectiveness could occur. What form would the experiential activities of a human being have, to have this property of autoprotective rigidity?

What must be the process in order for autoprotectiveness to occur?

The general form of the analysis of the autoprotective process will not be to present a process model and then show that it manifests autoprotectiveness. At best, that would simply show that autoprotectiveness is possible at the process level; it would provide a minimal sufficiency analysis of the autoprotectiveness of a process but would not reveal any necessary features of an autoprotective process. The analysis, accordingly, will focus on the properties that a process must have in order for it to manifest the functional property of autoprotectiveness. There will be two general parts to such an analysis: the first will concern itself with those process properties that are necessary to autoprotectiveness by virtue of being constitutive of it; the second will concern those properties that are necessary further manifestations of it.

<u>Centrality</u>

Centrality is a congnitive aspect of any autoprotective process. It is constitutively essential to autoprotectiveness, in that any process that is not central in the required sense cannot be autoprotective. The basic intuition of centrality is that any process that is subordinate in some sense to some other process will thereby be subject to evaluation and change from the perspective of that superordinate process--and will therefore <u>not</u> be autoprotective. By definition, the subordinate process cannot prevent the superordinate process from examining and potentially changing the nature of the subordinate process or of the superordinate-subordinate relationship. Centrality means that there is no superordinate process, no superordinate way of being, from which the given process can be examined and changed.

There are two basic senses of this superordinate relationship, and two corresponding aspects of centrality. The first is a functional centrality in the sense that the autoprotective process cannot be functionally subordinate to, cannot be a subroutine for, or a means toward, some other process. When means are not serving their ends well, they will tend to be changed, and thus not autoprotective. When change in such a case does not occur, then we must ask, "Why is this dysfunctionality persistent, rigid?" and we are back to the case of a derivative rigidity. An autoprotective process, then, cannot be functionally subordinate; conversely, it must be functionally central.

Functional means-ends relationships are a dominant way of thinking about human beings in this culture, but a much more fundamental characteristic of persons is epistemic reflexivity. An autoprotective way of being in the world must not only be functionally central, it must also be epistemically central. The critical point here is that we not only have goals that make use of their goals, processes that make use of other processes, but in the above functional sense we also have goals and processes that are _about_ other goals and processes, that reflect on them, goals and processes that have an epistemic, a knowing, relationahip with other goals and processes. The subordinate relationship here is not one of instrumental means to an end, but rather one of an epistemically instantiating or satisfying object (or process or condition or property or way of being). The superordinate _knows_ the subordinate, and the subordinate epistemically satisfies or fails to satisfy various criteria of the superordinate. Such an internal epistemic relationship is not commonly acknowledged or examined in psychology, but its reality cannot be denied (it is, for example, the foundation of developmental stages, of the knowledge of logical necessity, of higher reaches of human potentiality, etc.; Bickhard, 1978; Campbell and Bickhard, 1986). Such internally epistemic goals are generally called _values_. An autoprotective stance in the world, then, must be both functionally and epistemically central. In being epistemically central, it must involve the most central, the most deeply implicit, values of the person--the values that constitute the person, that are lived, not just espoused, by that person.

A corollary of this epistemic centrality with respect to values is that an autoprotective stance in the world must be central to a person's sense of self. A _person_ is an entire way of being in the world; a self is the "core" of that way of being. There have been and still are many differing attempts at explicating that intuition of the self as "core," but I suggest that a fundamental aspect of the self is that it is the core in precisely the epistemic sense explicated above. One's _self_ is precisely one's understanding of oneself, one's epistemic relationship to oneself. If the superficial circularity of this is troublesome, then it can be rendered more precisely, if somewhat more cumbersomely, as follows; A person's _self_ is that person's reflective understanding, is that person's internal organization of epistemic relationships, is that person's relationship to his or her highest epistemic level (core) values.

Autoprotectiveness, then, must involve a person's central sense of values about the self. Autoprotectiveness must be constituted at that central level of experiential process.

Terror

Centrality is a cognitive constitutive necessity for autoprotectiveness; terror is a roughly equivalent motivational necessity. The argument here concerns the nature of the "prevention of examination and change" that constitutes autoprotectiveness: centrality ensures that there is no current perspective from which the way of being could be changed; terror is what prevents such a higher-order perspective from becoming. To simply not have a current higher-order perspective on one's current way of being is a kind of incompleteness that is inevitable for everyone. It is a version of finiteness--one cannot have a higher-order perspective on one's current highest level. So, although centrality is necessary for autoprotectiveness, centrality itself must answer the question of rigidity: How can a central way of being be autoprotective? How can it "protect" its centrality? How can it prevent the development of a higher perspective?

Since there is no current higher order perspective, the issue is precisely the prevention of the development of one. A functionally central part of a self organizing system (a highest-level goal or end at the top of a hierarchy of means and ends) will control interactions of the system with the environment without itself being controlled by a still higher level: by hypothesis, there is no current higher level. But any such functionally central part of the system will have been constructed by the self organizing processes of the system and will be subject to change or may be superseded by further constructions of that self organizing process. Functional centrality is not at all the same thing as "self organizational centrality." The problem is to determine the properties of processes that can guide, and potentially misguide, self organization in a sense similar to that in which functional centrality guides interaction with the environment.

Functionally central parts of a system can guide learning, but only with respect to parts of the system that are subordinate to those central parts (the functionally central parts determine what counts as success and failure for the subordinate parts). They do not guide learning for themselves, however, and thus cannot protect their own centrality. Some sort of process is required that can guide the construction of even functionally central parts of the system.

Emotions have the required properties. Emotions clearly participate in the guidance of environmental interactions, but they also participate in the guidance of learning and development, of self-organization, including that of functionally central parts of the system. The additional key property of emotions in this regard is that emotions, among other things, not only provide heuristics for self-organization (as well as for interaction), but also provide heuristics that can guide "away from" as well as "toward." Experienced failures of even functionally central activities can invoke self-organization, and there is a sense in which the implicit success conditions for correcting those activities can be said to indirectly guide that self-organization, but these implicit guidances of unrepresented success conditions of functional centrality cannot guide <u>away</u> from anything. (Explicit learning heuristics can guide both toward and away, but these cannot be functionally central; they are intrinsically subordinate to the categorizations of problem types for which heuristics have been developed.) Negative emotions, however, can both guide self-organization and guide <u>away</u>, thus potentially participating in an autoprotective organization of processes, guiding away from what would be required for change. Negative emotions begin to capture the necessary self-organizational "centrality." With central values involving deep negative emotional aspects, we find a confluence of functional centrality, epistemic or reflective centrality, and self-organizational "centrality."

Autoprotectiveness requires avoidance not only at the level of interactive process, but also at the level of metaprocess, at the level of self-organization. Emotions have the necessary character to provide both, and it is thus emotions that must provide the motivational aspect of autoprotectiveness. Emotions yielding motivations to avoid are negative emotions, and thus an autoprotective stance involves negative emotions in the core central values concerning the self. Such negative emotions can involve disgust, contempt, dread, anger, and so on, but the most primitive negative emotions include distress, anxiety, and fear, with the extremes of panic and terror. I will use the word "terror" as a generic term for the primitive emotional motivation underlying autoprotectiveness, although all available terms seem to say both too much and too little for what is needed here. (That is, too much in that they are all construed in terms of fully explicit adult versions--the autoprotective emotion will in general be neither adult nor explicit--and too little in that they do not capture well the "core of one's being" sense of the autoprotective emotion--in that respect "dread" is a useful word, but its connotations are both too adult and too passive.) Autoprotectiveness, then, is constituted as a central terror at the center of, and concerning, one's being, one's self. Autoprotectiveness is a (cognitively) central (emotional) terror. Centrality and terror jointly constitute autoprotectiveness. Autoprotectiveness processes, however, will necessarily manifest a number of additional characteristics, some of which will be examined at this point.

<u>Self Confirming</u>

One important necessary manifestation of autoprotective rigidity is that the underlying terror will tend to elicit confirmations of that terror from others. That is, psychopathology will have a tendency to be engaged in cycles of self-fulfilling prophecy. These cycles, however, will not constitute the rigidity, but will rather be a manifestation of it, and will not be invariably present, but will rather be a tendency that is sometimes manifested.

The terror concerning the self may have the form of a terror concerning who or what I am, or what I might be, or what I might become, but, in any of these cases it will strongly constrain the way in which I present myself to others. (Most examples will be given in the first person because the coherence that is being illustrated and invoked is an experiential, meaningful coherence.) I will develop many ways of being with others to hide what I fear may be so, to compensate for it, to try to escape it, and so on. A terror concerning myself is a terror concerning some sense of inadequacy, actual or potential, as a human being. It is a terror concerning some sense of actual or threatened failure to live up to full human status. It is a terror concerning my worth to others with respect to my own deepest values. Such a terror will severely constrain and distort my presentations of self throughout my life.

But such constrained presentations of self, such distorted ways of being, presuppose precisely the inadequacies that I fear the most. Only with respect to such inadequacies would I engaged in such inadequate ways of being with others. My compensations and cover-ups thus implicitly communicate to others precisely what I want most desperately to hide, and define me to others in precisely those ways that I most fear to be defined. Others, in turn, will tend to pick up on these implicit self-definitions and respond "appropriately" to them, confirming my terror.

Such an interpersonal process are sometimes manifested in day-to-day interactions, but will be most likely to occur in deeper intimate relationships, in which more of the person is intrinsically involved, and thus the threat of exposure of what I fear is that much greater. Also, the confirming response from the other is not always as certain nor as clear as it would be in the pure self-fulfilling prophecy case. The other will have his or her own idiosyncracies, strengths and weaknesses, fears and sensitivities, and so on, but the distortions of the pathological individual's way of being are inherently not as fulfilling to others as if those distortions were not present, and the almost inevitable negative reactions of some form to those distortions will be experienced as confirming the fundamental sense of inadequacy.

Autoprotectiveness presents my being as precisely what I fear I might be (or am) and thus tends to elicit "appropriate" confirming responses from others.

Self-Affirming

Distortions in an individual's way of being will not only tend to elicit negative reactions from others, thus seemingly confirming the underlying terror, but they will also tend to result in an even more fundamental form of reflexive support for that terror. The distortions of my way of being are potentially as available to me as they are to others. My being so kind to women, for example, so as to compensate for my felt terror of being fundamentally weak and pathetic, is something that I "know" for the weak and pathetic attempt to be humanly attractive that it "really" is. My way of being presupposes my terror and thus affirms its truth. After all, only someone who was truly inadequate would go about with all of the distortions and compensations and avoidances that I find in myself. Autoprotectiveness as a way of being affirms precisely what I am terrified I might become or already be.

Self-Constituting

Autoprotectiveness is not only self-confirming and self-affirming, it is most fundamentally self-constituting. It not only indicates via others' and my own reactions that I am what I fear, it constitutes me precisely as what I fear. The terror of inadequacy distorts and constrains my construction of myself, distorts the development of my self, perhaps, from, early childhood. The terror of inadequacy, the sense of awfulness about myself, distorts not only the way I present myself, but also who I have come to be. The presuppositions of my being who I am are precisely what I most fear. Only someone who is in fact what I am terrified of being can in fact be as I am. Autoprotectiveness constitutes me as what I am terrified I might be (or am). My attempts at coping with a central terror of inadequacy and weakness have constituted me as a person of distortions, compensations, and avoidances; and those distortions, compensations, and avoidances at the center of my life and living *are* weakness and inadequacy--a weak and inadequate person *is* one who lives such a not fully human existence.

The realization of these points, especially the last, in therapy can be truly terrifying, in very much an explicit, adult sense. To acknowledge, examine, and explore them is to acknowledge, examine, and explore the truth of my worst terrors about my being. It is to contradict the entirety of the self that I have constructed in order to avoid and compensate for that terror of inadequacy. It feels like losing that self, annihilating the way of being that I am, for it is to give up on the struggle against the terror that I have formed myself around. It is to face the felt certainty of the devastating human inadequacy. It is to ultimately acknowledge my basic failure to *be* a human being. Such an examination is extremely difficult, in both a cognitive and a motivational sense, yet only by such a process can those terrors, and concomitant distortions, be transcended. Only by giving up the struggle against the terror can the rigidity of that struggle be overcome, but the struggle cannot be transcended without directly confronting its felt truth and the senses in which it is *in fact* true. Only by giving up that struggle can the rigidity be overcome, but only by understanding that struggle can it be given up. Only by understanding what it is that I am doing that constitutes that struggle (phenomenologically, experientially doing, doing in terms of interpretations of meanings and values, "certainly" doing, not merely behaviorally doing) do I have the choice to do something different, and thus step outside of the struggle. The near impossibility of that confrontation is precisely constitutive of autoprotective rigidity.

To even approach such a confrontation can be exceedingly difficult. To focus on the central terror is to be distracted from my focus on the continuous struggle of compensation. This can seem pointless, in that my central inadequacy is simply my reality; it is what I have to live with, to accommodate to, to compensate for. It can be frightening, in that distraction from my compensations reduces their effectiveness, exposing my inadequacies of potential and rendering them even more real. It can be terrifying, in that it risks giving up the compensatory struggle altogether, which would be, as I anticipate it, to sink totally into my centrally terrifying inadequacy: I cannot conceive that my central terror is something that I am doing and can therefore do differently; it seems to me that it _is_ reality, and the only way I can conceive of losing it would be to fool myself, to dupe myself, concerning the reality of those inadequacies. In this way, the very conception of giving up on the compensatory struggle can feel like giving up on the self, giving up on serving the self in the best, the only, way that seems possible. It can feel like a giving up on myself and my life as worth serving with the efforts of my compensations. The only sense of worth and value and self respect that I do have, for example, may come from my sense of honesty and integrity in holding the values that I know I do not, and intrinsically cannot, fulfill or the "honesty" and "integrity" of castigating and deprecating myself, for those failures are themselves my only source of self-respect. In this way, the possibility of freeing myself can come to feel like a betrayal or abandonment of myself, so long as the sense of inadequacy is taken as an immutable given rather than as a consequence of my activity.

At still another level, the idea of transcending a central terror and thereby giving up on the derivative and compensatory struggles can simply seem incomprehensible, because those "compensations" are the problems of living (for me). They constitute my understanding of the boundaries and the issues of life, at least for me if not for others. They are what I want help with; I want to be able to engage in them more effectively. To "give up" on them makes no sense. In this version I do not understand them as deriving from any central terror at all, but rather as being immutably definitive of my self and of the basic issues of life and living.

Self Double Bind

Autoprotectiveness is constituted most fundamentally as a centrality of a terror concerning the self. It also manifests the properties of being self-confirming, self-affirming, and self-constitutive. There are in addition a number of other aspects of an autoprotective way of being, some of which make connections with other discussions of psychopathology.

One important additional property of autoprotectiveness is that it manifests the logical property of being an internal, self-directed double bind. "Double bind" is sometimes used in a loose sense to refer to any contradictory imperatives or expectations, but the intent here involves the strict sense of "double bind" in which the fact of a message or directive contradicts the content of the message or directive.

The autoprotective terror involves a directive concerning the avoidance of whatever inadequacy the terror is about, but that presumed inadequacy is an inadequacy of the person holding the terror. The terror is a directive to the individual to not (fully) be his or her self, lest that terror-laden inadequacy become realized and manifest. The autoprotective stance, then, is constituted as a directive to not be oneself, to not be who one really is. But being who one is, is the only thing that anyone can possibly do, and yet the autoprotective directive itself is part of who the rigid individual is. So being who one is, is in part to be directing oneself not to be who he or she is--a deep double bind concerning one's basic being.

Double binds generally have the form of some version of "be spontaneous" (be spontaneously happy, or sensitive, or caring, or authoritative, etc.), but this version is particularly virulent: being spontaneously not spontaneous is being who you really are! For to be spontaneously who you really are is to sink fully into the inadequacy, while to be not spontaneous in your evasions, distortions, and compensations, is to fail in your struggle against that inadequacy. Double binds as usually considered are also social in nature, while this one is intrinsically intrapersonal. Interpersonal or intrapersonal, the only escape from a double bind is to transcend the framework within which it is posed. For the autoprotective double bind, that framework is constituted in the central self terror, and transcending it requires confronting it.

Self-Contradiction

The internal double bind of the autoprotective person is a self imperative not to be oneself. There is a converse of this, in that the rigid process is being exactly what it is denying of itself. That is, I deny my worth, my value, my legitimacy in my compensations, avoidances, cover-ups, apologies, and distortions. I affirm my lack of humanness in fleeing from myself, in my self-constitution, in my very living of my self-denial. But precisely in so affirming my lack of humanness, I affirm my legitimacy in declaring myself illegitimate, my value in judging myself worthless, my power in making myself weak. I must be of value in order that my judgment of valuelessness have any value; I must be powerful in order that my self-constitution and presentation as powerless have any power; I must be of worth in order that my deprecations of unworthiness have any worth. Precisely, my self-constitution as powerless, illegitimate, and valueless is itself an assertion, a presumption, a self-constitution as powerful, legitimate, and worthy.

When the autoprotective individual realizes that he is the one, or she is the one, who is making all these central terrors true, then the terrors are no longer experienced as an external truth about oneself, a given about one's being that must be "accepted" and to which one must be accommodated. Instead, they can come to be realized as something that one is doing, and therefore as, something that one can do differently. My being in the world as a weak and illegitimate being is instantiating its power and legitimacy precisely in those constitutions and affirmations. If I can come to understand the power that I am exercising in constituting my weakness, then I can have the freedom to choose to constitute myself differently. Such a realization is one powerful manner in which an individual can transcend an internal terror.

External Contradiction

My compensations, distortions, and evasions are for myself, but they are in large part to others. They are self-presentations, masks, to the world in an attempt to escape the consequences of my true inadequacies and live instead in terms of those desperate fakeries. They are attempts to induce the world to treat me as being adequate and human, to induce unawareness of, reassurances about, compensations for, and denials of my core failings. This is an externalization of the self contradiction. Such a way of being is a social living out of being so powerless as to have to ask others for my power, so empty of meaning as to have to ask others for my meaning, so illegitimate as to have to ask others for my legitimacy, and so on for my worth, my adequacy, my basic humanness. The implicit request in this aspect of rigidity already constitutes me as not being what I am requesting.

External Double Bind

Simultaneously, This way of being imposes a double bind on the other, in that I am asking him or her to accept me, to judge me, to declare me to be adequate and fully human, and yet the acknowledgment that I need such acceptance, judgment, or declaration is an acknowledgement that I am not adequate or fully human. I put the other in a position of either failing to respond to my request or of contradicting that response in the very act of responding.

External Power

The rigid personality is forbidden from being fully himself or herself. The central "truth" about the rigid personality is that it is fundamentally inadequate to cope with the foundational human issues of worth, meaning, purpose, and so on. The rigid individual cannot survive these issues alone, so he or she must depend on some other power to be able to live with them, must rely on some "not-self" way of being to be strong enough to avoid their threat. The avoidances, compensations, and distortions constitute the person's reliance upon such an external power for living. More basically, those avoidances, compensations, and distortions constitute that individual's sense of a felt "non-self" way of being that is more powerful, capable, worthy, attractive, and meaningful than one is oneself. In this sense, autoprotectiveness intrinsically involves a reliance upon an external "non-self" power for living (E. Becker, 1973). Its implicitly involves a "deal" with life that an external power be so right, powerful, good, or whatever is required that one can "succeed" in life by virtue of holding fast to that power, of living up to that deal, even though one's self, per se, is unworthy and inadequate.

<u>Lack of Courage</u>

The terror of one's inadequacy, the double binding self-directive not to be oneself, the sometimes desperate reliance upon an external power, all constitute a terror of being oneself, of even acknowledging oneself. They all constitute a lack of courage for living, a lack of courage in the face of the seemingly overwhelming problems of life with respect to that which is fundamentally inadequate (A. Adler, 1964; M. Bickhard and B. Ford, 1976; 1979).

<u>Cosmic Loneliness</u>

An autoprotective central terror is a sense of the inadequacy of my deepest being to fulfill my own most central values and senses of the meaning of living. It is a kind of void, an emptiness, in the center of my being. It is this void that makes me less than fully human. It is this void that I seek to fill with others, or to hide from others, or to compensate for in being with others. The central inadequacy is a central emptiness, a differentness, a less-than-oneness from "everyone else," from all the full human beings in the world.

Such a central void is a sense of the barrenness of my being. It is an aloneness, an isolation from meaningfulness and fulfillment. There is an intrinsic loneliness in this feeling, in that by definition no one could possibly want to make true contact with me in that barrenness, no one could genuinely accept that emptiness and inadequacy. But there is an even deeper aloneness, and a consequent cosmic loneliness, in that full human beings do not <u>have</u> such a void. There is not only no one who would be with me in my emptiness; there is no one (fully human) with whom I share the experience, the awfulness, of that emptiness. I am cosmically alone in my very aloneness. I am cosmically lonely in my barren loneliness.

It is this deep sense of emptiness and "unwholeness" as a human being that H. Kohut and object relations theorists seem to be exploring (Eagle, 1984; Greenberg and Mitchell, 1983). H. Guntrip's example of the woman who dreamed that she "opened a locked steel drawer and inside was a tiny naked baby with wide open expressionless eyes, staring at nothing" (1973, p. 152) is a deep expression of such a core barren isolation. If the model that I am presenting is correct, however, then such a core terror is central to all psychopathology, not just to particular schizoid or borderline types of psychopathology. Such a view seems to be partially emerging in the psychoanalytic literature, though it is far from consensual (Eagle, 1984).

Finitude

A central sense of inadequacy, of terror concerning the self in facing living, is a sense of finitude in the face of the infinite demands of life. One's finitude in confrontation with the intrinsically infinite demands for omniscience and omnipotence in living, the demands for never failing in being a full human, in being an ethical being, in being worthy, in making the best decisions in one's life, in being strong enough, or attractive enough, or tough enough, is a finitude that guarantees inadequacy. A finite being cannot know enough, cannot do enough, cannot understand enough, cannot consider enough, to fulfill such infinite values and their demands. Finitude is a fundamental existential aspect of being human, and, therefore, so is inadequacy in the face of infinite life demands.

The inadequacy of finitude is a basic truth in any central terror, but it is this existentially certain finitude that grounds the sense of barrenness, of less than humanness, of aloneness. It is a sense of finitude that seems to separate me from all others, that degrades me below humanity. It is in this finitude that I feel most alone, and cosmically alone in having a being that is finite.

Finitude, however, is an aspect of being for everyone. It is most deeply in my finitude that I feel most different from, most separated from, most inadequate with respect to others, and yet it is precisely in my finitude that I am most like everyone else, that I am potentially most sharing with others, that I am least alone. It is in owning the weakness of my finitude that I am most strong, in accepting the illegitimacy of my finitude that I am most legitimate, in acknowledging the unworthiness of my finitude that I am most worthy, and in embracing the intrinsic inadequacy for human contact of my finitude that I am most human, most a full human being, most together with all humanity. The deepest fundamental fact of an autoprotective central terror, the intrinsic finitude of human existence, is simultaneously the truth that transcends the terror.

The Elite

The full human beings in the world may be everyone else besides me; or they may be only some special elite, who do (in my eyes) live up to my, to the central, values (an elite that I fail to be a full member of); or that elite may be formed of people with some special powers of judgment concerning those values. If I meet a member of my elite in this sense, I may have an intense need for acceptance, for affirmation, by such a person. I may need to be accepted into the membership of those who are cool, or cultured, or tough, or smart, or intellectual, or "together," or popular, or "deep," or who never let anyone get the better of them, or whatever, or I may need to be accepted as a man by a woman, or as a woman by a man, or as a parent by my children, or as worthy by a hero or mentor, and so on. More deeply, I may live in abject terror of rejection, by that person, which would confirm all of my most horrible fears about myself. I become a supplicant. I may even find myself bound to the terror of possible rejection by someone I don't even like or respect, as long as in some sense I have given them a power of judgment with respect to my central being.

Fragility

Affirmation from others can feel very good with respect to the central terror, but it can never satisfy. The very act of affirmation is a contradiction of the content of the affirmation. The response to the double bind that I impose on others (at least on members of my personal elite) is turned back on me in their response to it. Consequently, no affirmation does anything more than hold off the terror for a while. It doesn't constitute me any differently; it doesn't change the terror--it simply soothes it. Consequently, my fundamental sense of inadequacy and vulnerability remains.

Furthermore, any such reassurances that I do receive are invalidated because they are simply responses to my masks, my fakery, my pleadings, my compensations. They are not really about me; no one knows me enough for them to be truly about me. My desperation makes any positive judgment impossible to receive because it is always, at least potentially, an insincere, deluded, or pitying response to that desperation itself (or its manifestations). Still further, any temporary reassurance that I do feel simply affirms that I am so weak and inadequate as to need such soothing.

Conversely, my fear of another's judgment of my inadequacy is ever present and overwhelming, for I "know" how true such a judgment would be. It would penetrate to the core of my being. I am deeply vigilant for such possible confirmations of my inadequacy. I am vigilant even for the absence of explicit reassurances and reaffirmations. Such an absence, even a short absence, can give me a deep anxiety that I have been "truly" seen and judged for my "true" inadequacy. So my need for reassurance may be constant and effectively unsatisfiable, and my awareness of that unsatisfiability can give me just one more affirmation and constitution of my inadequacy. My sense of well being, when and to the degree to which it is possible for me to have such a sense, is massively vulnerable and fragile.

Inauthenticity

When one's way of being in the world intrinsically denies and forbids one's way of being in the world, it is not possible for that being to be full and open and honest and genuinely spontaneous. To be self-contradicting is to be constrained and distorted. The self-imperative to be not oneself and the reliance on an external power are forms of fleeing from oneself, of denying oneself. An authentic openness and resoluteness of one's central self values and meanings is not possible for someone who is attempting to live an evasion, an annihilation, of that central self. The rigid personality cannot be authentic (C. B. Guignon, 1983; M. Heidegger, 1962; J. L. Mahta, 1976).

The concept of autoprotectiveness makes contact with a number of aspects of psychopathology discussed in the current literature. I have briefly indicated connections with self-fulfilling prophecies, Becker's external powers, deals with life, Alfred Adler's lack of courage, and the existentialist finitude and inauthenticity. Each of these could be given much more extensive elaboration and exemplification, and there are other possible connections as well. The general point that I would like to draw from these examples, however, can already be made: The connections are all with aspects of the process of psychopathology. That is, autoprotectiveness has been argued to be the basic functional characteristic that constitutes psychopathological processes as being, in fact, rigidly pathological. The general discussion has shown, in addition, that any autoprotective process will also manifest a number of other aspects of the psychopathological process that have been noted in the literature.

CONCLUSION

This chapter proposes the abandonment of the substance-structural ontology for human beings that is fundamental to standard discussions of psychopathology. One example of the rare exceptions to such standard presuppositions is R. Schafer (1976), although I have basic disagreements with the model he presents. In this chapter an experiential process ontology is proposed in which the fundamental conceptual problem shifts from how to cause change to how to free from rigidity. In an open process system rigidity requires an autoprotective process, which in turn can be instantiated only in the form of central self value terrors. Such a model of autoprotectiveness connects with a number of other process characteristics of psychopathology noted in the literature, such as self fulfilling prophecy, internal double binds, reliance on external powers, a lack of courage in living, and inauthenticity.

There are a number of further questions that this discussion immediately gives rise to that, because of space limitations, cannot be addressed here. For example, why is it that core terrors are rarely directly encountered in therapy? One reason is that therapy most commonly, and necessarily so, deals with distorted functioning in the world that is _derivative_ from core autoprotectivenesses rather than from core terrors per se. A second reason is that clients are only occasionally aware of their core terrors. This, of course, raises the question of what is the status of those core rigidities, with the obvious standard answer being that they are "unconscious." I argue that such an answer is deeply inadequate, and I propose an alternative model to account for truths about a person that are not phenomenologically available to that person. A second obviously pertinent question would be, "What are the implications of this model for therapy?" Again, there is not space for the reasoning or elaboration; the quick answers are that therapy is intrinsically relational (rather, than, for example, interpretational) and that therapy is intrinsically ethical (rather than just being an activity to which ethics applies). I raise such questions at this point primarily to acknowledge their relevance and importance. Any serious attempts at addressing them await later writings.

There would seem to be at least two levels of implications involved in this chapter: one concerning the specific results with respect to psychopathology and psychotherapy, and the other concerning the importance and productivity of taking one's ontological assumptions and commitments seriously. Clearly, I urge both. But whatever the specific deficiencies of the analysis of psychopathology might be perceived to be, it seems more than clear that the general questions of rigidity and structures, and the even more general issues of ontological assumptions and commitments, require serious attention. With rare exceptions, they remain presupposed and unexamined.

REFERENCES

Adler, A. 1964. Social Interest. New York: Capricorn.

Becker, E. 1973. The Denial of Death. New York: Free Press.

Bickhard, M. H. 1978. "The Nature of Developmental Stages." Human Development, 21: 217-33.

Bickhard, M. H., R. L. Cooper, and P. Mace. 1985. "Vestiges of Logical Positivism." Human Development, 28, no. 5: 240-58.

Bickhard, M. H., and B. Ford. 1976. "Adler's Concept of Social Interest: A Critical Explication." Journal of Individual Psychology, 32: no. 2: 27-49.

Bickhard, M. H., and B. Ford. 1979. "Subjective Adaptationalism: An Adlerian Metapsychology." Journal of Individual Psychology, 35, no. 2: 162-86.

Campbell, R. L., and M. H. Bickhard. 1986. Knowing Levels and Developmental Stages. Basel: Karger.

Eagle, M. 1984. Recent Developments in Psychoanalysis. New York: McGraw-Hill.

Gendlin, G. 1970. "A Theory of Personality Change." In J. Hart and T. Tominson, eds. New Directions in Client-centered Therapy. New York: Houghton.

Greenberg, J., and S. Mitchell. 1983. Object Relations in Psychoanalytic Theory. Cambridge, Mass.: Harvard University Press.

Guignon, C. B. 1983. Heidegger and the Problem of Knowledge. Indianapolis: Hackett.
Guntrip, H. 1973. Psychoanalytic Theory, Therapy, and the Self. New York: Basic Books.
Heidegger, M. 1962. Being and Time. New York: Harper and Row.
Mahta, J. L. 1976. Martin Heidegger: The Way and the Vision. Honolulu: University of Hawaii Press.
Schafer, R. 1976. A New Language for Psychoanalysis. New Haven: Yale University Press.
Shapiro, D. 1981. Autonomy and Rigid Character. New York: Basic Books.
Suppe, F. 1973. "Theories, Their Formulations, and the Operational Imperative." Synthèse, 25: 129-64.
Wachtel, P. L. 1977. Psychoanalysis and Behavior Therapy. New York: Basic Books.

8

Eclecticism and Integration in Psychotherapy

Sol Garfield

In this chapter, several of the important developments in the field of psychotherapy and behavior change are discussed, including the relative decline in popularity of psychodynamic orientations and the increase in eclectic preferences. The variation in operational meanings of an eclectic approach is described, and possible commonalities among diverse forms of psychotherapy are suggested. In terms of patients' views of the important factors in psychotherapy, the characteristics of therapists and some common aspects of therapy appear to be emphasized over differences in techniques. Finally, some of the recent emphases on convergence and integration in psychotherapy are discussed.

In the past 40 years some rather unusual and surprising changes have occurred within the field of psychotherapy and behavior change. In the 1940s and 1950s the field was clearly dominated by psychoanalysis and psychodynamic emphases. Although several other approaches were available to psychotherapists, these had little apparent impact (Garfield, 1981). In fact, the influence of the model of long term "intensive" psychodynamic psychotherapy was so pronounced that other and briefer therapies were looked down upon as superficial, symptom-oriented, "supportive," and essentially inferior forms of psychotherapy. In a survey of members of the Division of Clinical Psychology of the American Psychological Association conducted in 1960, E. L. Kelly (1961) found that 41 percent indicated that they adhered to a psychodynamic orientation. This was the single most popular theoretical orientation, although, surprisingly, about 40 percent of the respondents classified themselves as eclectic. Less than 10 percent claimed a preference for learning theory or behavioral theory.

The high frequency of psychodynamic preference in Kelly's (1961) survey was not surprising. What was somewhat unanticipated, perhaps, was the number of clinical psychologists who indicated that they were eclectic. I was quite intrigued by these findings and some 14 years later attempted to conduct a comparable study. In that investigation, R. Kurtz and I found that some interesting changes in theoretical preference had taken place (Garfield & Kurtz, 1976). With a new sample, a noticeable decline was evident in the preference for a psychodynamic orientation from 41 percent to 19 percent. However, in this later survey, approximately 55 percent of the respondents identified themselves as eclectic. Thus, by the mid-1970s it seemed that a significant change had occurred in theoretical preferences and that the psychodynamic approaches had declined markedly in popularity, at least among clinical psychologists. The percentage selecting a behavioral orientation increased 1 percentage point, to about 10 percent. These findings, by the way, are quite similar to those reported by Kelly, L. R. Goldberg, D. W. Fiske, and J. M. Kilkowski (1978) in their 25-year follow-up of U. S. Veterans Administration trainees. In their study, 58 percent of their subjects indicated an eclectic orientation, as compared to 17 percent who specified a psychodynamic (psychoanalytic, neo-Freudian, or Sullivanian) orientation.

The changes in theoretical preference probably reflect some dissatisfaction with the once dominant psychodynamic approaches to clinical intervention. One may hypothesize also that some dissatisfaction with prevailing therapeutic approaches was reflected in yet another unpredictable development, the proliferation of therapeutic schools. The spirit of American free enterprise was evident in the way new psychotherapeutic schools and approaches emerged. In the early 1960s, for my own edification and amusement, I compiled a list of over 60 different forms and types of psychotherapy. Some years later, a publication from the National Institute of Mental Health (NIMH) made reference to 130 different forms of psychotherapy (Report of the Research Task Force of the National Institute of Mental Health, 1975), and a more recent publication mentions over 200 varieties of psychotherapy (Hesink, 1980).

Psychotherapy, it appeared, had become a growth industry.

We have thus experienced a decline in the importance of the previously most influential and dominant forms of psychotherapy and have witnessed the accompanying surge of eclectism and proliferation of therapeutic schools. In addition, more recently, another possible development has been visible, even if its manifestations are still somewhat limited. Here I refer to some writings and presentations discussing convergence or integration in psychotherapy (Goldfried, 1980, 1982; Gurman, 1981; Marmor and Woods, 1980; Wachtel, 1977). The present series of articles also is a manifestation of this trend. I have interpreted all of these different developments as reflecting, at least to some degree, a lack of satisfaction with the current approaches and orientations within the field of psychotherapy and behavior change. This clearly is a personal view. However, individuals who are truly satisfied with a particular approach usually do not go seeking or developing a different approach, nor would they necessarily become eclectic, convergent, or integrationist if this were so. Dissatisfaction with current procedures leads therapists to change loyalties or to experiment in some way with attempts to modify or enlarge their existing approach to psychotherapy.

In some instances, individuals may lay claim to inventing or developing a "new" therapeutic approach, although some of these new approaches actually can be discerned in the writings of ancient philosophers and sages. Most therapists, however, sincerely try to incorporate aspects of different therapies that they believe allow them to better and more efficiently meet the needs of their patients or clients. Such individuals are usually viewed as practicing eclecticism, although recently the more dignified "convergence" or "integration" have been used.

ECLECTICISM

Although the term eclectic has tended to be viewed rather negatively by a number of individuals, as being synonymous with "muddle-headedness" or minimal brain damage, it is surprising that so many clinicians have admitted that they are eclectic in their work. Eclecticism is perceived as adherence to a nonsystematic and rather haphazard clinical approach. Theoretical purity, on the other hand, provides the clinician with an organized system for dealing with personality and behavioral problems, a rationale, and some sense of security. In addition, predictions derived from theoretical constructs supposedly can be tested, and allow for revising the theory in the light of new data. Such advancement in knowledge, however, cannot be expected from the more subjective and less organized eclectic approaches. Although there is some truth to such statements, they do not necessarily tell the whole story.

Individuals who adhere closely to one theoretical view tend to have both restricted vision and selective perception. If such individuals do not outgrow their single orientation in the normal process of maturation, they may be manifesting what Freud termed a fixation. Any theoretical view in psychology or psychotherapy reflects one conceptualization of the area or processes involved, and to the extent that it is a partial view, the individual who adheres exclusively to one specific orientation is bound to be neglecting phenomena that are not considered or glossed over as inconsequential from that point of view. As I see it, the price of theoretical purity is the exclusion of variables the theory does not emphasize or overlooks.

Those who follow an eclectic course also pay a price for doing so. I am tempted to say that the cost is "overinclusion," but this term has been used so frequently in studies of patients diagnosed as cases of schizophrenia that I must refrain from doing so. A large number of therapists have become eclectic because of dissatisfaction with one therapeutic approach. Their attempts at eclectic psychotherapy are for the most part idiosyncratic and nonsystematic (Garfield and Kurtz, 1977). Such individuals, depending upon their past training and experience, may try out various procedures and combine them in their own way. Many of these clinicians stated that their eclectic efforts represented an attempt to individualize their therapy in order to better meet the needs of their patients. In a real sense, perhaps, they were attempting to adhere to a dictionary definition of the term eclectic, which is, "choosing what appears to be best from diverse sources, systems, or styles" (American Heritage Dictionary, 1971). If this accurately describes an eclectic approach, it does not seem too productive to criticize it, for who really wants to oppose "choosing what appears to be best"?

The matter, however, is not that simple, for the dictionary does not really tell you what being an eclectic psychotherapist means or what individual eclectic therapists actually do, operationally and therapeutically speaking. In our study of eclectics, we found that there were 32 different theoretical combinations used by 145 eclectic psychologists, and these appeared to be blended and used in individually unique ways. In the absence of clear guidelines, theoretical or otherwise, possibly more procedures were used than were necessary, and perhaps the most efficient and effective procedures were not always utilized. Unfortunately, we have no data on this matter, but only conjecture.

Thus, two possible limitations of an eclectic approach are evident. It does not represent a single operationalized approach, but rather can be used to designate any combination of therapeutic procedures. Consequently, it lacks specificity, and this limits the adequate description of the therapy. A second limitation, which follows from the above, is the difficulty involved in evaluating such a variable therapy. Although an eclectic approach allows the therapist greater flexibility and access to a wider range of procedures than is the case of most other therapies, it is nonsystematic, covers a multitude of sins, and is difficult to evaluate. What choice, therefore, does the poor therapist have? Let us postpone a discussion of this issue and consider some other aspects of therapy that may be pertinent to the overall issues discussed.

DIFFERENCES AND COMMONALITIES IN PSYCHOTHERAPY AND BEHAVIOR CHANGE

Although there has been a tendency to emphasize the differences among psychotherapeutic approaches, both theoretically and procedurally (Binder et al., 1976; Morse and Watson, 1977), a few individuals have pointed to at least some possible common factors or commonalities among the diverse psychotherapies. Since I have discussed this matter in some detail elsewhere (Garfield, 1980), my treatment here will be brief.

An early influence on my own thinking was the phenomenon that all of the supposedly different forms of psychotherapy claimed to be effective. Not one of them was modest enough to claim to be less effective than the others, even though most had not been evaluated adequately. Now, if all of the different therapies are successful, how does one account for this phenomenon? Are the therapies really different? Do all roads actually lead to Rome? Are some therapies more effective with certain kinds of clinical problems than others? With the possible exception of behavioral therapies, most psychotherapies have been claimed to be what I have termed "universal therapies," ready and able to cure all sorts of psychological maladies. Is it possible that the positive results claimed by all of the psychotherapies are due, at least in part, to their reliance on common factors that are operative in all the psychotherapeutic approaches?

Stimulated also by the early writings of S. Rosenzweig (1936), and M. Levine (1948) and by the study reported by R. W. Heine (1953), I began to consider the idea of common factors with some seriousness and made reference to them in my 1957 clinical psychology textbook and again in the 1974 version (Garfield, 1957, 1974a). However, until fairly recently, such views received relatively little attention. Jerome D. Frank and his colleagues did call attention to "nonspecific" factors, factors that influenced outcome but were not specific to any particular form of psychotherapy (Frank, 1973; Stone et al., 1966). However, such factors tended to be viewed as superficial and relatively unimportant, or as contaminating variables in research on psychotherapy (Kazdin and Wilcoxon, 1976). Thus, although they received recognition, particularly from researchers, they were not usually viewed as crucial variables in psychotherapy. Frank (1971) and E. F. Torrey (1972), however, did publish papers that clearly discussed common factors potentially evident in most of the psychotherapies, as being of some consequence in the outcomes secured.

Some obvious reasons explain why many individuals may not respond positively to the proposition that there may be a number of, common factors operating in psychotherapy and that these may account for at least an important part of the changes relating from therapy. Such a view detracts from the importance and "truth" of their own approaches, and as Frank has mentioned, an old Chinese maxim states that "a wise man does not question the source of his well-being." Clearly, an emphasis on common factors dilutes or diminishes the uniqueness of established schools of psychotherapy and even calls into question some of the basic doctrines and beliefs of their adherents. My interest in such factors, however, was basically to understand and then to hypothesize some potential variables that may actually facilitate change, regardless of how they are viewed or evaluated from the perspective of diverse schools of psychotherapy (Garfield, 1980). Thus the expectations that a client had concerning therapy might be one such common variable. Since most forms of psychotherapy involve a dyadic relationship, the perceptions that each of the participants has toward the other might also influence the process and outcome of psychotherapy. If the client perceived the therapist as an interested, knowledgeable, competent, and nonjudgmental person, the chances for positive outcome would appear to be enhanced. Conversely, if the therapist were perceived in an opposite fashion, the probabilities of successful outcome would appear to be diminished, regardless of the therapist's particular orientation. In a similar way, a number of other possible common factors or variables might come into play in psychotherapy that would have some potentially positive impact on therapeutic progress, but that would tend to go unrecognized or to receive little attention or emphasis. Such aspects of therapy as giving the patient an explanation for his or her difficulties, providing some support and reassurance, encouraging and reinforcing desirable behaviors, allowing the opportunity for emotional release, and several others, are some of the common factors that have been suggested in this regard (Garfield, 1980).

Although the probable importance of common factors in psychotherapy may appear plausible to me and to others, little systematic research exists on many of the hypothesized common factors. Client expectations have received a moderate amount of research investigation, with at least some positive results, although such findings are far from conclusive or uniform (Bootzin and Lick, 1979; Kazdin and Wilcoxon, 1976; Lick and Bootzin, 1975; Morgan, 1973; Wilkins, 1971, 1973, 1979). The hypothesized variables are not well defined as yet and certainly must be viewed tentatively. Nevertheless, there are research data from comparative studies of outcome in psychotherapy that are at least consistent with the general hypothesis of common variables operating in different forms of psychotherapy.

J. E. Meltzoff and M. Kornreich (1970), in their comparative review of students, concluded that "there is no current evidence that one traditional method is more successful than another in modifying psychopathology, alleviating symptoms or improving adjustment" (p. 200). H. B. Roback (1971), in a review of selected studies, found no difference in reported outcome between behavior therapies and insight therapies. A similar finding as to the lack of superiority of one form of psychotherapy over another has been reported in the reviews by Allen E. Bergin and M. J. Lambert (1978) and by I. Luborsky, G. Singer, and L. Luborsky (1975).

The study by R. B. Sloane and his colleagues comparing psychodynamically oriented psychotherapy with behavior therapy also did not secure significant differences in outcome between the two forms of therapy. Comparable findings were reported by L. C. Miller and others (1972) in comparing analytic and behavior therapy in children. Studies comparing systematic desensitization with implosion or flooding also have not always reported consistent findings concerning the relative efficacy of these two forms of therapy (Gelder et al., 1973).

A few additional reviews that compared outcome in different types or forms of psychotherapy can also be referred to here. Three reviews that compared time-limited, or brief, psychotherapies with time-unlimited therapies also reported comparable results for these types of psychotherapy. Two of the reviews primarily evaluated research on individual therapy (Butcher and Koss, 1978; Luborsky et al., 1975), whereas the other compared brief and unlimited marital and family therapies (Gurman and Kniskern, 1978). Finally, reference can be made to the analysis of over 400 studies of outcome in psychotherapy by M. L. Smith, G. V. Glass, and T. I. Miller (1980) utilizing meta-analysis. As many of you are aware, their analyses did not reveal much in the way of important differences among a variety of forms of psychotherapy.

Thus, the bulk of the evidence comparing different forms of psychotherapy and behavior change indicates a surprising lack of difference among the forms evaluated. Admittedly, one can criticize many of the studies conducted, as well as the reviews that have attempted to analyze and evaluate portions of these studies (Kazdin and Wilson, 1978; Rachman and Wilson, 1980). There are, to be sure, some studies that suggest that specific behavioral procedures are more efficacious than some other approaches for selected disorders. These studies might also be faulted on some counts, but this is of relatively little consequence for our present discussion. Even if the findings from such studies are valid, behavioral therapies could consist of both common and specific therapeutic variables (Garfield, 1980). A large number of studies, however, do appear to lend support to the view of comparability of outcome among different forms of therapy, and this to me suggests the possibility and plausibility of common factors operating in these different forms of psychotherapy. Although, as noted, this view is not well received by a number of psychotherapists, there is another consideration that makes me feel it is a reasonable one.

Although adherents of a particular school of psychotherapy tend to emphasize its particular approach and its distinctly unique aspects, their descriptions of their therapy may not (and frequently do not) correspond to their actual behaviors and interactions in the therapeutic situation. As E. Glover (1955) and others have shown (Lieberman et al., 1973), therapists of particular schools or orientations actually function and view therapeutic phenomena in different ways. Therapists from different schools may also show similar qualities and behaviors in their work with patients. H. L. Lennard and A. Bernstein (1960), in their analysis of psychotherapy as a social system, stated:

> that despite major differences in the outlook and the behavior of each therapist and each patient, there are major similarities among therapist-patient pairs in terms of the way the interaction unfolds. . . . This finding raises many questions for those who tend to stress differences between therapists in their theoretical orientation and who overemphasize the importance of the "school" to which a therapist belongs as the determinant for what transpires during therapy. . . . The enormous amount of similarity in the therapeutic systems suggests to us that what is shared by different therapist-patient pairs may be at least as therapeutic as that which is unique (pp. 193-94).

A somewhat similar observation was offered by C. I. Barrett, I. E. Hampe, and L. C. Miller (1978) in their review of research on psychotherapy with children:

> It would seem redundant to state that reciprocal inhibition therapy and play

> therapy are two different techniques. To a large extent, though, the activities conducted under these two names are quite similar, so much so that. . . we found it possible and profitable to describe a generic set of procedures that we found ourselves using no matter what kind of treatment we were using. Moreover, these common procedures probably accounted for the fact that we obtained no deferential effect. One treatment was the other (p. 431).

Thus, while some observers have noted possible commonalities among different forms of therapy, adherents of particular approaches believe that their forms of therapy are different and, of course, better than other forms. However, it is the actual behaviors of the therapists, and not just their theoretical orientation, that influence the process and outcome of therapy, and therapists may be unaware of some of the behaviors and thus fail to acknowledge their possible significance of them. Variables of possible importance may not be considered by therapists, if they are not conceptualized as important features of their particular orientation. Most therapists probably tend to see what they anticipate seeing in terms of their theoretical perspective, and researchers study the variables of theoretical importance to the particular systems under investigation. Analysts and psychodynamic therapists do not emphasize such simple and nondynamic interactions as suggestion, reassurance, and encouragement, but are such therapists' interventions never manifested in these therapies? Should all the credit for positive client change go to interpretation and insight? Behavior therapists have not really emphasized such client-centered therapeutic conditions as empathy, self-congruence, and depth of interpersonal exploration, but as indicated in the study by Sloane and others (1975), the behavior therapists were certainly not deficient in the manifestations of such conditions. Carl R. Rogers never emphasized verbal reinforcement as a variable in client-centered therapy, but his use of reinforcement was illustrated in two separate studies of his taped therapy interviews (E. J. Murray, 1956; C. B. Truax, 1966). Cognitive therapists emphasize cognition, but does this mean that this is all there is to their therapeutic approach and their interactions with their clients? Do they never make use of assigned tasks, homework assignments, reinforcement, behavioral rehearsal, and other procedures? Actually, as we know, they in part do (P. C. Kendall and S. D. Hollon, 1979).

In a related manner, I would also like to refer to the reported observations of the therapy conducted by two well known therapists, J. Wolpe and A. A. Lazarus. Several observers devoted five days each to such observation, and their comments are interesting and pertinent to the present discussion (M. H. Klein et al., 1969). "Perhaps the most striking impression we came away with was of how much use behavior therapists make of suggestion and of how much the patient's expectations and attitudes are manipulated" (p. 262).

These observers also emphasized the important discrepancies they noted between the stated theoretical orientation of behavior therapy and the actual implementation of the therapy. Thus, for example, they point out that while overt behavior is emphasized, the behavior therapist usually has to deal with "the patient's report of that behavior." I believe similar kinds of comments could be made about other forms of therapy, and it is to the credit of Wolpe and Lazarus that they exposed their therapy to scrutiny by observers with other orientations.

PATIENTS' VIEWS OF PSYCHOTHERAPY

On the basis of what has been presented thus far, it seems reasonable to hypothesize that therapists may use procedures that are not emphasized theoretically or otherwise highlighted in their form of therapy, and that possible factors common to many, if not most, varieties of psychotherapy are operative. Furthermore, a number of research studies do not show different results for different forms of therapy; the existence of common therapeutic factors may account in large part for such findings. A final point to be made here is that therapists generally explain or account for the variables leading to positive outcome from their own perspective and tend to emphasize their own particular techniques (Feifel and Eels, 1963). Patients, however, tend to view their experience in psychotherapy somewhat differently. As indicated in the study by Sloane and others (1975), the patients in both therapy groups who had positive outcomes tended to ascribe their improvement to more or less the same factors. These included the following:

1. The personality of your doctor.
2. His or her helping you to understand your problem.
3. Encouraging you gradually to practice facing the things that bother you.
4. Being able to talk to an understanding person.
5. Helping you to understand yourself. (p. 206)

Clearly, as pointed out by these investigators, practically all of these items "can be classified as 'encouragement, advice, or reassurance, factors common to both behavior therapy and psychotherapy. None of the items regarded as very important by the majority of either group of patients described techniques specific to one therapy" (Sloane et al., 1975, p. 207).

Somewhat similar findings have been reported by others (Heine, 1953, Feifel and Eels, 1963) in studies of more traditional nonbehavioral therapy, and in a study of patients who received behavior therapy, V. L. Ryan and M. N. Gizynski (1971) also reported similar findings. According to them, the patients in their study "felt, and the authors would agree, that the most universally helpful elements of their experience were the therapist's calm, sympathetic listening, support and approval, advice and faith" (p. 8). Although most behavior therapists may not stress such variables as the important ones in their therapy, from the perspective of the patient, the situation is apparently different.

From my own perspective these kinds of findings are extremely interesting and potentially important. The factors stressed by patients as the important variables in their therapeutic progress are variables that appear to be common to most forms of psychotherapy and that also receive comparatively little emphasis in most of the psychotherapies. Although we are dealing here with the perceptions and evaluations of patients, rather than with some more objective appraisal of the therapeutic process, it is important to give serious attention to such responses. After all, a person's view of reality is largely mediated and governed by his or her perceptions. The fact that many patients who undergo different forms of psychotherapy mention similar therapeutic variables as being the ones that are important cannot be disregarded. Although this finding can be interpreted in different ways, the consequences appear to be similar. On the one hand, it is possible that many differently designated psychotherapies use a number of similar procedures or interactions that have an impact on the client, but that these are not emphasized or particularly attended to in the formal accounts of the therapy. As has been mentioned already, the therapist, whether analyst or behaviorist, may exert a therapeutic effect by his or her confidence in the therapy, calmness, interest in the client, encouragement, explanation, and the like. However, to many therapists, these are just relatively minor aspects of therapy that are really not worth talking about. On the other hand, and I do not view these two aspects as mutually exclusive, it is possible that observably different procedures or interactions are perceived similarly by patients and have comparable or similar impact. For example, modeling, systematic desensitization, and implosion are procedurally different. However, the patient's positive response to these diverse procedures may be due, at least in part, to positive expectations about the treatment; belief in the rationale provided; trust in a sympathetic, knowledgeable, and confident therapist; and the actual confronting of the fear-producing stimulus. I have selected behavioral techniques for illustrative purposes, but other therapies can easily be substituted.

Although adhering to one theoretical system provides a more consistent rationale and set of guidelines for the therapist than is true for the eclectic therapist, it does have its limitations. Potentially positive features and procedures of other therapeutic approaches may not be used, and there is a greater likelihood that the patient may be forced to adjust to the therapy offered, rather than that the therapeutic procedures are selected in terms of optimal treatment for the patient's difficulties. Furthermore, as I have suggested here, common factors that may be operative in therapy are overlooked, and a more correct view of the therapeutic process is neglected. We must go beyond the variables postulated by any given approach and study the actual behaviors and interactions that take place between therapist and client, and their impact on the client. Research along these lines may not only suggest factors that appear to be common among diverse forms of psychotherapy, but may also increase our knowledge of those variables that actually play an important role in facilitating change (Garfield, 1974b). In this way, a more meaningful and effective eclectic form of therapy may result.

CONVERGENCE, INTEGRATION, AND ECLECTICISM

Recently, as noted earlier, there has appeared to be what might be termed an ecumenical movement in psychotherapy. One aspect of this has been the attempt by several psychotherapists with psychodynamic or behavioral orientations to combine these two very different approaches in a number of ways. Paul L. Wachtel's (1977) book attempted such an integration, and more recently, J. Marmor and S. M. Woods (1980) published an edited volume of previously published articles on the same general topic. Several articles have reported individual and unique attempts to combine or integrate psychodynamic and behavioral approaches (L. Birk and A. W. Brinkley-Birk, 1974; B. W. Feather and J. M. Rhoads, 1972; J. Marmor, 1971). Various kinds of combinations have been described, including the use of two separate therapists, one from each orientation (R. T. Segraves and R. C. Smith, 1976), and the use of systematic desensitization with the patient's drive-related imagery underlying the avoidance behavior (B. W. Feather and J. M. Rhoads, 1972). Behavior therapists have appeared to broaden their therapeutic perspective by acknowledging the importance of the relationship in psychotherapy. An article by M. R. Goldfried (1980) indicated that a number of therapists, including several prominent behavior therapists, have indicated a dissatisfaction with narrow sectarianism in psychotherapy and a need for a broader outlook. A. A. Lazarus (1977) has indicated a similar view. A 1979 survey (G. E. Swan) also found that a number of behavior therapists indicated an eclectic orientation. What becomes of all these different manifestations of possible rapprochement, integration, or eclecticism, remains to be seen. However, more than ever before, there does appear to be a greater awareness of the limitations of adhering strictly to one therapeutic orientation and a desire to look further for additional psychotherapeutic principles and procedures.

The fact that some well known individuals who have been identified with particular orientations have expressed such views toward integration and convergence is a positive sign. However, to simply combine existing theoretical views or to add some behavioral techniques to a psychoanalytic orientation will not represent any major advance. Such "integration" is likely to be limited by the theoretical orientations retained or emphasized. The resulting conglomerate, in keeping the original concepts and explanations of the previous approaches would hinder, I believe, the process of ascertaining what is truly therapeutic in the various systems of psychotherapy. In my view, we have to go further, and one important step in the desired direction is to delineate and operationalize some of the common variables that seem to play a role in most psychotherapies and, perhaps, to regard them as a basis for a clearer delineation of psychotherapeutic principles and procedures. This may not be popular, but I think it will be worth the effort.

REFERENCES

American Heritage Dictionary of the English Language. 1971. New York: American Heritage.

Barrett, C. I., I. E. Hampe, and L. Miller. C. 1978. "Research on Psychotherapy with Children." In S. L. Garfield and A. E. Bergin, eds. Handbook of Psychotherapy and Behavior Change. 2nd ed. New York: Wiley.

Bergin, A. E., and M. J. Lambert. 1978. "The Evaluation of Therapeutic Outcomes." In S. L. Garfield and A. E. Bergin, eds. Handbook of Psychotherapy and Behavior Change. 2nd ed. New York: Wiley.

Binder, V., A. Binder and B. Rimland. 1976. Modern Therapies. Englewood Cliffs, N.J.: Prentice-Hall.

Birk, L., and A. W. Brinkley-Birk. 1974. "Psychoanalysis and behavior therapy." American Journal of Psychiatry, 131: 499-509.

Bootzin, R. B., and J. R. Lick. 1979. "Expectancies in Therapy Research: Interpretive Artifact or Mediating Mechanisms?" Journal of Consulting and Clinical Psychology, 47: 852-55.

Butcher, J. N., and M. P. Koss. 1978. "Research on Brief and Crisis-oriented Therapies." In S. L. Garfield and A. E. Bergin, eds. Handbook of Psychotherapy and Behavior Change. 2nd ed. New York: Wiley.

Feather, B. W., and J. M. Rhoads. 1972. "Psychodynamic Behavior Therapy: Theory and Rationale." Archives of General Psychiatry, 26: 496-502.

Feifel, H., and J. Eels. 1962. "Patients and Therapists Assess the Same Psychotherapy." Journal of Consulting Psychology, 27: 310-18.

Frank J. D. 1971. "Therapeutic Factors in Psychotherapy." American Journal of Psychotherapy, 25: 350-61.

Frank, J. D. 1973. Persuasion and Healing. 2nd ed. Baltimore: Johns Hopkins University Press.
Garfield, S. L. 1957. Introductory Clinical Psychology. New York: Macmillan.
Garfield, S. L. 1974a. Clinical Psychology: The Study of Personality and Behavior. Chicago: Aldine.
Garfield, S. L. 1974b. "What Are the Therapeutic Variables in Psychotherapy?" Psychotherapy and Psychosomatices, 24: 372-78.
Garfield, S. L. 1980. Psychotherapy: An Eclectic Approach. New York: Wiley.
Garfield, S. L. 1981. "Psychotherapy: A 40-Year Appraisal." American Psychologist, 36: 174-83.
Garfield, S. L., and R. Kurtz. "Clinical Psychologists in the 1970s." American Psychologist, 31: 1-9.
Garfield, S. L., and R. Kurtz. 1977. "A Study of Eclectic Views." Journal of Consulting and Clinical Psychology, 45: 78-83.
Gelder, M. G., J. H. Bancroft, D. H. Gath, D. W. Johnston, A. M. Mathews, and P. M. Shaw. 1973. "Specific and Non-Specific Factors in Behavior Therapy." The British Journal of Psychiatry, 123: 445-62.
Glover, E. 1955. The Technique of Psychoanalysis. New York: International Universities Press.
Goldfried, M. R. 1980. "Toward the Delineation of Therapeutic Change Principles." American Psychologist, 35: 991-99.
Goldfreid, M. R., ed. 1982. Converging Themes in Psychotherapy. New York: Springer.
Goldfried, M. R., and G. C. Davison. 1976. Clinical Behavior Therapy. New York: Holt, Rinehart, and Winston.
Gurman, A. S. 1981. "Integrative Marital Therapy: Toward the Development of an Interpersonal Approach." In S. H. Budman, ed. Forms of Brief Therapy. New York: Guilford.
Gurman, A. S. and D. P. Kniskern. 1978. "Research on Marital and Family Therapy: Progress, Perspective and Prospect." In S. L. Garfield and A. E. Bergin eds. Handbook of Psychotherapy and Behavior Change. 2nd ed. New York: Wiley.
Heine, R. W. 1953. "A Comparison of Patients' Reports on Psychotherapeutic Experience with Psychonanlytic, Nondirective and Adlerian Therapists." American Journal of Psychotherapy, 7: 16-23.
Hesink, R. ed. 1980. The Psychotherapy Handbook: The A to Z Guide to More than 250 Different

Therapies in Use Today. New York: Meridan, New American Library.

Kazdin, A. E., and L. A. Wilcoxon. 1976. "Systematic Desensitization and Nonspecific Treatment Effects: A Methodological Evaluation." Psychological Bulletin, 83: 729-58.

Kazdin, A. E., and G. T. Wilson. Evaluation of Behavior Therapy: Issues Evidence, and Research Evidence. Cambridge, Mass.: Ballinger.

Kelly, E. L. 1961. "Clinical Psychology-1960: Report of Survey Findings." Newsletter. Division of Clinical Psychology, Winter, pp. 1-2.

Kelly, E. L., L. R. Goldberg, D. W. Fiske, and Kilkowski, J. M. 1978. "Twenty-Five Years Later. A Follow-up Study of the Graduate Students in Clinical Psychology Assessed in the VA Selection Research Project." American Psychologist, 33: 746-55.

Kendall, P. C. and S. D. Hollon eds. 1979. Cognitive-Behavioral Interventions: Theory, Research, and Procedures. New York: Academic Press.

Klein, M. H., A. T. Dittman, M. B. Parloff and M. M. Gill. 1969. "Behavior Therapy: Observations and Reflections." Journal of Consulting and Clinical Psychology, 33: 259-66.

Lazarus, A. A. 1977. "Has Behavior Therapy Outlived Its Usefulness?" American Psychologist, 32: 550-54.

Lennard, H. L. and A. Bernstein. 1960. The Anatomy of Psychotherapy: A System of Communication and Expectation. New York: Columbia University Press.

Levine, M. 1948. Psychotherapy in Medical Practice. New York: Macmillan.

Lick, J. R. and R. R. Bootzin. 1975. "Expectancy Factors in the Treatment of Fear: Methodological and Theoretical Issues." Psychological Bulletin, 82: 917-31.

Lieberman, M. A., I. D. Yalom, and M. B. Miles. 1973. Encounter Groups: First Facts. New York: Basic Books.

Luborsky, I., B. Singer, and L. Luborsky. 1975. "Comparative Studies of Psychotherapies: Is It True that 'Everyone Has Won and All Must Have Prizes'?" Archives of General Psychiatry, 32: 995-1007.

Marmor, J. 1976. "Dynamic Psychotherapy and Behavior Therapy. Are They Irreconcilable?" Archives of General Psychiatry, 24: 22-28.

Marmor, J., and S. M. Woods eds. 1980. The Interface between the Psychodynamic and Behavioral Therapies. New York: Plenum.
Meltzoff, J. E., and M. Kornreich. Research in Psychotherapy. New York: Atherton.
Miller, L. G., C. I. Barrett, I. E. Hampe, and H. Noble, 1972. "Comparison of Reciprocal Inhibition, Psychotherapy and Waiting List Control for Phobic Children." Journal of Abnormal Psychology, 79: 269-79.
Morgan, W. G. 1973. "Nonneccessary Conditions or Useful Procedures in Desensitization: A Reply to Wilkins." Psychological Bulletin, 79: 373-75.
Morse, S. J., and R. I. Watson, Jr. 1977 Psychotherapies. A Comparative Casebook. New York: Holt, Rinehart and Winston.
Murray, E. J. 1956. "A Content-Analysis Method for Studying Psychotherapy." Psychological Monographs, 70 (13 whole no. 420).
Rachman, S. J., and G. T. Wilson. 1980. The Effects of Psychological Therapy. 2nd ed. New York: Pergamon. Report of the Research Task Force of the National Institute of Mental Health. Research in the Service of Mental Health. HEW Publication no. (ADM) 75-236. Rockville, MD: HEW, 1975.
Roback, H. B. 1971. "The Comparative Influence of Insight and Non-Insight Psychotherapies on Therapeutic Outcome: A Review of the Experimental Literature." Psychotherapy: Theory, Research and Practice, 8: 23-25.
Rosenzweig, S. 1936. "Some Implicit Common Factors in Diverse Methods of Psychotherapy." American Journal of Orthopsychiatry, 6: 412-15.
Ryan, V. L., and M. N. Gizynski. 1971. "Behavior Therapy in Retrospect: Patients' Feelings about Their Behavior Therapies." Journal of Consulting and Clinical Psychology, 37: 1-9.
Segraves, R. T. and R. C. Smith. 1976. "Concurrent Psychotherapy and Behavior Therapy: Treatment of Psychoneurotic Outpatients." Archives of General Psychiatry, 33: 756-63.
Sloane, R. B., F. R. Staples, A. H. Cristol, N. J. Yorkston, and K. Whipple. 1975. Psychotherapy Versus Behavior Therapy. Cambridge, Mass.: Harvard University Press.
Smith, M. L., G. V. Glass, and T. I. Miller. 1980. The Benefits of Psychotherapy. Baltimore: Johns Hopkins University Press.
Stone, A. R., S. D. Imber and J. D. Frank. 1966. "The Role of Non-Specific Factors in Short-Term

Psychotherapy." American Journal of Psychology, 18: 210-17.
Swan, G. E. 1979. "On the Structure of Eclecticism: Cluster Analysis of Eclectic Behavior Therapists." Professional Psychology, 10: 732-39.
Torrey, E. F. 1972. "What Western Psychotherapists Can Learn from Witchdoctors." American Journal of Orthopsychiatry, 42: 69-76.
Truax, C. B. 1966. "Reinforcement and Nonreinforcement in Rogerian Psychotherapy." Journal of Abnormal Psychology, 71: 1-9.
Wachtel, P. L. 1977. Psychoanalysis and Behavior Therapy: Toward an Integration. New York: Basic Books.
Wilkins, W. 1971. "Desensitization: Social and Cognitive Factors Underlying the Effectiveness of Wolpe's Procedure." Psychological Bulletin, 76: 311-17.
Wilkins, W. 1973. "Expectancy of Therapeutic Gain: An Empirical and Conceptual Critique." Journal of Consulting and Clinical Psychology, 40: 69-77.
Wilkins, W. 1979. "Expectancies in Therapy Research: Discriminating among Heterogeneous Non-Specifics." Journal of Consulting and Clinical Psychology, 47: 837-845.
Wilson, G. T. and I. M. Evans. 1977. "The Therapist-Client Relationship in Behavior Therapy." In A. S. Gurman and A. M. Razin eds. Effective Psychotherapy: A Handbook of Research. New York: Pergamon.

9

Hypnosis: An Overview of a Modern Fairy Tale

Maryanne Galvin

It has been my pleasure and good fortune to present my chapter "Clinical Hypnosis: Origins, Myths, and Applications" in a South American culture so rich in history, mysticism, legend, and lore. Given this scenario, this chapter will build on the metaphor of fairy tales and their ecumenical appeal.

Structurally, fairy tales are typically divided into six segments that develop throughout:

1. The beginning
2. The people involved
3. Exposition of the problem-defined (the trouble, trying to understand it)
4. The ups and downs of the story
5. The climax
6. Catastrophe (Lysis)

THE BEGINNING

"Once upon a time . . ." All good tales begin somewhere in a far off land and time. The hypnosis tale has its early origins in both the Old and New Testaments. The use of early hypnotic techniques with children originated in ancient times.

Accounts of sick children responding to healing methods based on suggestion and faith are noted in the Bible (I Kings VIII: 17-24; Mark X: 17-22). Children in primitive cultures have employed trance phenomena in initiation rites and other ceremonies (Mead, 1949).

Primitive people have long resorted to dancing, chanting, and singing to drive away demons and restore health. Ancient Greeks used special rooms for "temple sleep" to create a sense of well-being, and throughout other cultures, references have been made to visions, the magic touch, and exorcism as means of healing.

THE PEOPLE

The modern history of hypnosis begins with Franz Mesmer, an Austrian physician whose interest in the healing power of magnetic influence was a mystical extension of the attention to magnetic forces among astronomers and physicists of that time. In 1766 Mesmer wrote a dissertation, "The Influences of the Planets on the Human Body" (Tinterow, 1970). He enjoyed a wide following until the King of France appointed a commission to evaluate "animal magnetism." That commission, comprised of Chairman Benjamin Franklin, the astronomer A. Bailly, Chemes T. Lavoisier, and J. Guillotin, among others, found that mesmerism did not work but that the results were dependent upon the imagination of the patient. The professional community lost respect for mesmerism, and few physicians continued to use it.

James Braid, a Scottish physician, revived mesmerism, giving it the name "hypnosis," yet disbelief regarding its efficacy in treatment persisted. Jean-Martin Charcot and Sigmund Freud (Tinterow, 1970) both were interested in its application, but Freud ceased to use it because all patients "could not be hypnotized" (Tinterow, 1970). William McDougall brought interest to the use of hypnosis as a means of treating shell-shocked soldiers in World War I, and John Watkins used hypnotic principles in the treatment of war neuroses in World War II.

Perhaps most recognized as a genius in the application of hypnosis to medicine and psychotherapy was Milton H. Erickson. As a tribute to his work, a post humous "birthday," the International Congress on Ericksonian Approaches to Hypnosis and Psychotherapy, in December 1980, attracted the largest gathering ever in the world of professionals who use hypnosis. Hypnosis does lay claim to being one of the most scientific and systematic ways to approach the field of psychotherapy.

And so, the historical groundwork and the people involved have been set to continue the unraveling of events in the hypno-tale.

THE EXPOSITION

There exist several misconceptions about hypnosis. It is not a state of unconsciousness. It will not weaken the mind. People do not do in hypnosis things they would not do otherwise. The person in a state of hypnosis will not be "lost" if something happens to the hypnotist. Hypnosis is also not a panacea (Wolfberg, 1972).

What then is hypnosis? Although derived from the Greek hypnos, meaning sleep, it is not sleep. There does not seem to be a singly accepted definition of hypnosis, and controversy exists as to whether it is a state of consciousness or whether a person possesses a trait of hypnotic responsiveness. Most clinicians accept both positions. That is; people differ in their hypnotic responsiveness, and those who are highly hypnotizable choose when to experience the hypnotic state.)

The "trance state" is the state of aroused attentive focal concentration with diminished peripheral awareness. The analogy that seems most fitting here is that hypnosis helps people to fixate onto the visual system. We have two kinds of vision: we have "macular," or "focal," vision and "peripheral vision." Macular vision is intense, it is full of color but it is rather narrow in field. One can only see with one eye fixation with any detail in color and an arc of about five to seven degrees. Within that arc, one can see a great deal of detail and color, but outside of it, vision and the acuity with which one can see falls off dramatically. The only way we maintain a detailed environment is by constantly shifting our gaze.

The trance state is analogous to macular vision; it is intense and detailed, but it lacks that view of the periphery. Our ordinary awareness is more like peripheral vision; it is not as detailed and intense, but it enables us to cover a variety of information. For example, my hope is that you are so enthralled right now that you are not noticing the sensations of your back resting against the chair or your bottom settled onto the seat of the chair; those are sensations that are in service of focusing on something else. This could be referred to as a "dissociative state."

This is not to say that this is a trance experience, but it is analogous to a trance state. It is similar to the experience of being at a play or a movie and being so enveloped in it that you feel you are part of the movie or play, not part of the audience, and that you are "jolted" when the piece ends. It is then that you realize "Oh, yes, . . . here I am at the theater and I must get a taxi to get home." The notion of being so absorbed in your experience that you lose your ordinary scanning awareness is the trance-like experience. Recent data indicate that people who are capable of having such trance-like experiences are also highly "hypnotizable." The crucial issue is this intense focused concentration and the ability to suspend critical judgment and peripheral awareness. That is the essence of the hypnotic trance experience. Along with the focal concentration is an interpersonal process referred to as the "compulsive triad". Because one is focusing so intently, there is a tendency to suspend conscious critical judgment, and that allows an interesting triad of events to occur. Amnesia and rationalization are also hallmarks of the triad. These consistently occur in everyday life. It is rare for us to do things for reasons that are crystal clear. How often do we know why we are complying, have no amnesia at all for the reason behind our behavior, and are not, to some extent, rationalizing? One great French anthropologist said that "myths are things that never were true but always will be."

THE UPS AND DOWNS

There are a number of persistent myths about hypnosis that tend to cause confusion in the field of psychotherapy. To clarify definitions within the realm of hypnosis, I shall examine in greater depth ten of the most prevalent myths and supply a glossary of common terms, which will take us from induction to arm levitation.

Myth 1: Hypnosis is Sleep

Braid thought hypnosis was a form of "nervous sleep." He borrowed that concept from D. Shakow, who felt that the trance stare was pathological sleep. In examining a person in trance, superficially one might think the client asleep. This is probably best understood by observing persons who are in a state of hypnosis and by listening to their descriptions of the experience. Generally, clients close their eyes, their respiration rate slows, and their muscles relax, but that is where the similarity to sleep ends. Other hypnotic phenomena may occur differently, depending upon the depth of trance. When clients are asked to describe the experience, they usually note mental and physical relaxation. Some call it the most profound relaxation they have ever known, and one client likened it to "feeling like chopped liver."

Furthermore, by electroencephalogram criteria, the trance state is the opposite of sleep. If anything, the "alpha" state will show itself. That is, hypnosis activates the "noise" the brain makes when it is resting but alert. So the trance state is the opposite of sleep. E. R. Hilgard and J. R. Hilgard (1975) did an interesting experiment using the Stanford Hypnotic Susceptibility Scale with a group of students who were peddling on an exercycle. This group received scores as high as those of the control group, which was given the test in a serene, restful atmosphere. One is awake and alert in trance.

Myth 2: Hypnosis is Projected onto a Client

The image to work with here involves an old Svengale and Trilby movie from late-night television. The basic plot has a sad-sack girl with no voice who is hypnotized and made to be a great operatic star. It would be more accurate to frame this event as the girl being highly hypnotizable and coached by Svengale. One "projects" nothing onto the client. The skill of the facilitator or therapist is in assessing the client's ability to respond. Similar to doing a Babinski, one does not take pride in whether the toe goes up or down. The pride is derived in being able to elicit the sign and make use of its meaning. This model is most appropriate for inducing hypnosis.

Myth 3: Only Weak-minded or Sick People are Hypnotizable

If anything, the opposite is true. This was a subject of great debate in the last century between the rival schools of the Sal Petrierre, where Shakow resided, and H. Bernheim's department at Nancy. Bernheim took the position that hypnotizability was actually a capacity of normal, healthy people. It appears in reviewing his reports that he had to take that position. Unlike Shakow, he was hypnotizing his staff, and if he had reached the same conclusion that they were all suffering from nervous sleep, he would have had very few people working for him. Nonetheless, history does bear him out.

Myth 4: Hypnosis Occurs Only When a Practitioner Decides to Use It

My hunch is that each person reading this chapter has used hypnosis at one time or another. An example from clinical practice will demonstrate this point. A general practitioner had a young woman in our clinic who suffered from pathological hiccough. He taught her some breathing exercises and the hiccough stopped. Then, a few years later, they started again. The physician was about to retire and move to Florida. He agreed to see her before his departure, and again he taught her the breathing exercises, she practiced them, and the hiccough ceased. Fifteen years later she went to see a well known psychiatrist because her symptoms had started again. He taught her self-hypnosis. He called the general practitioner in Florida and asked how he had learned to use self-hypnosis so well. This inquiry elicited a rage response from the general practitioner who declared he would "never deal with the quackery of hypnosis." What he had essentially taught her was to restructure her experience and her physical tension with the hiccough.

If a surgeon making rounds were to say, "Good morning, Mrs. Jones, and how is your pain today?", some inpatients would constitute an instruction that in order to comply and be in tune with their doctor they had better have pain. The point here is: As psychotherapists, we must be aware of the spontaneous trance, a self-induced state of hypnosis that often occurs in psychotherapy and in daily living. Clients have that faraway expression, the eyes being fixed, unmoving, or having a glassy stare. They appear quiet, have a smoothing of face, lag in responding to your interaction with them, or perhaps make short, repetitive movements, such as nodding the head. As a therapist, the stage is set for you to deepen that experience and perform psychotherapy within a different medium. More discussion regarding altered states of consciousness will follow.

Myth 5: Hypnosis is Dangerous

One could take the position that it is far more

dangerous not to recognize when hypnotic phenomena are taking place than to systematically assess them. The descriptions provided earlier in this chapter regarding ideomotor relaxation responses should provide a cursory framework. More elaboration of the terms used to describe trance phenomena will be provided in the glossary.

Myth 6: Hypnosis is Questionable Therapy

There are varying points of view regarding the term "hypnotherapy." Hypnosis is an ancillary tool in the service of a primary discipline. As a psychologist, your discipline usually involves formulating a goal in treatment. The major point is in knowing how to assess a client, how to formulate a strategy that makes sense, and how to teach it to the client so that it is used in problem solving. Here is where the professional training enters. Steven Lankton and C. Lankton (1983) have developed well integrated models for interspersed hypnotic work with individuals, families, and groups. A careful review of the Lankton work will provide a bridge for the existing gap between schools of thought on "hypnotherapy" versus the rest of the world.

Myth 7: Symptom Removal Means Development of a New Symptom

One may assume that this grew from Freud's being influenced by the primary science of his day, just as we are by the primary sciences of today. However, his physics, primarily hydrolysis, raised questions in the "application" stage of reasoning. That is, his notion that if there was an underlying pressure caused by two conflicting unconscious forces and one were to remove the symptoms, this would allow for some disruption of this delicate balance and, lo and behold, another symptom would emerge. To this day this is true of pressure in hydraulics systems; however, it is not true in mental systems. We have overwhelming evidence in both the hypnosis and behavior therapy literature and in brief systemic therapy that when clients overcome a symptom in a respectable way, they feel so ebullient that they may overcome other symptoms in the manner of a "ripple effect." A line of reasoning to refute this myth might proceed as follows: It is true that if one were to coerce or deceive a client or have a strong expectation that the elimination of a symptom would lead to a new symptom, the client might well comply. However if one were to use hypnosis to help a client relieve himself or herself of a symptom and during therapy caused a new symptom, that would be a rationalization for therapeutic impotency.

Using Ralph Greensen's notion of developing a working alliance, it has been my observation that my best psychotherapy has been with clients who came to me initially for help with one "symptom" and "got over it". They then said, in essence: (1) "I see you can help me"; (2) "I am curious about why this happened"; or (3) "I have other related problems in my life and I want to explore them."

If anything, symptom-oriented work enhances motivation for long term psychotherapy if it is indicated. Or if it is not, the client can go past the symptom or presenting problem and move on. A general rule of thumb derived from Erickson is: Do the simplest things first. If it works, good. If it does not, that may also be a good way to begin psychotherapy. For instance, one young woman came to me for help loosing weight. She did initially loose a small amount and I asked her to return for a follow-up a year later and to speak to a group of graduate students in psychology about her experience. She aptly responded, "You <u>know</u> it didn't work!". She came and was prompted to tell them whatever happened. Her saga went as follows: "Well, I started doing the exercises the way you taught me--the breathing--and I lost ten pounds in the first two weeks. Then I started overeating again and began to wonder <u>why</u> I don't take better care of myself."

In many ways, the problem and solution became symbols in her cognitive structure for other aspects of her life. She continued, "I decided some group therapy might help and found that in many aspects of my life I wasn't taking care of myself!". Six months later she took off the rest of the weight, kept it off, and was afraid I would view this as a failure for hypnosis. <u>Au contraire</u>. Later in this chapter, aspects of restructured experiences will be delineated.

Myth 8: Women are More Hypnotizable Than Men

If ever there was an example of equality it is here. Now that "hypnotizability" is assumed to be a sign of relative psychological strength, men and women tend to be equally ranked.

Myth 9: Hypnotist Must Be Charismatic, Unique, or Weird

You may or may not have formed an impression of me, but rest assured, if you were to attend meetings of two professional associations that use hypnosis, dentists and psychologist/psychiatrists, (Hartland, 1971) you might never have see a more mundane group of people. For every person like Erickson, who would wear purple as Mesmer did, you will find a hundred who are as mainstream as Wall Street.

Myth 10: Hypnosis is Only a Superficial Psychological Phenomenon

In fact, hypnosis is a tool for exploring the mind-brain interface. In a sense, hypnosis is the opposite of psychotropic medication. Using psychotropic medication, one completes a physical manipulation to result in a change in psychological experiences. Using hypnosis, a psychological manipulation evokes a change in physical experience, from positive and negative hallucinations to alterations in sensory perception and motor control in various parts of the body. Thus, hypnosis can be a fascinating tool for exploring the mind-brain interface.

THE CLIMAX

Milton H. Erickson, M. D., earned a reputation for developing a clinical hypnosis and strategic psychotherapy that was highly creative and effective. Erickson's work has catapulted family therapy and various schools of psychotherapy into changes, large and small (Zeig, 1980). His influence has served to reshape the very way some clinicians think about their clients and problems.

Basically, his approach creates a planned therapeutic impact at several levels of human systems:

1. unconscious patterning and experiences;
2. conscious beliefs and frames of reference;
3. communications and social roles; and
4. family organizational structure.

Erickson's theory of intervention allowed him to cut through differences created by divergent theories of individual personality and family structure. Erickson's work has been applied to the clinical interview via the work of Lankton and Lankton (1983) and several other outstanding professionals.

I will now detail the premises regarding Altered States of Consciousness (ASCs).

Universal Existence of Altered States

In all cultures, people find it necessary to alternate between various discrete states of consciousness, even in normal daily activities. J. C. Pearce (1974) describes cultural rituals, rules, and artifacts that constitute methods for proper, and often distinctive, inductions of the altered states of consciousness.

Resources and Limits in Altered States

Imposition within particular states of consciousness limits the potentialities of available resources. Other resources are to be found in the ASCs. Any individual will experience alteration of discrete states in the course of daily activities. These will be described as mood, angles, feelings, and processes such as wondering, daydreaming, reflecting, and analyzing. Inherent in these groupings are possibilities for problem-solving interactions with the environment. Even young children have been taught to systematically attend to various changes in their states of awareness to best facilitate problem-solving potentialities (Galvin, 1983).

Functions of Altered States of Consciousness

Altering awareness, although unique to each individual, permits original combinations of the learning and experiences required in different life situations. Part of the natural problem-solving process involves shifting between these discrete angles, moods, sides, and frames (Galvin, 1983). Selecting and utilizing a particular ASC brings a specific set of discrete resources to the forefront.

Necessity of Shifting Between Different States

Each altered state produces a novel solution to a problem because the patterns and mechanisms that operate within us organize experiences in different ways. People need to alter their state to optimally interact with their environments. For example, the harried investments broker, after working hard for hours in a particular ASC (stabilized by caffeine and other stimuli from the office environment), goes out for a high powered game of tennis, or a two-martini lunch. How frequently does it happen that solutions to problems are conceived in these and other contexts? Furthermore, close examination would suggest that different states of consciousness are induced and stabilized within each of the "new" contexts.

Learning to Structure Altered States

Learning theory suggests that altering and stabilizing consciousness occurs in any skill (playing the piano, skating, handwriting). These activities can be performed well and efficaciously or randomly and inappropriately. It is assumed that people will structure and stabilize the ASC they consider to be most beneficial. Attempts will be made to induce or stabilize it in the most efficient manner. For instance, if a child abuser retrieves most of the resources he needs in an ASC that is characteristically associated with a certain level of tension, judgmental internal dialogue, a particular breathing pattern, and a limited range of voice tone, he or she will interact selectively with the social and physical environment so as to perceive opportunities to further stabilize the ASC. His employment of overly clumsy mechanisms of stabilization will strain the mechanisms and lower the operational quality of his performance. In other words, in these situations the abuser may resort to shouting, striking, and other abuse. Likewise, the function of some symptoms may be to continue the ASC that the symptom induces and stabilizes.

Social Induction and Stabilization

People get others to help structure a preferred and normal, daily ASC. Social systems, such as families, stabilize each member's preferred ASC or get other members to act so as to help stabilize their own state. Members interact so as to maneuver other members into assisting the stabilization process. This may be accomplished by shared agreements on beliefs, rituals, and experiences, or it may be done by resorting to ulterior and defensive behavior (Laing, 1972).

The induction of ASCs is done by means of conscious playful maneuvers, seduction, manipulation, courtship, childrearing, and so on, and by means of unconscious automatic strategies, defenses, and repetitive "game" sequences, as well as by means of daily transactions.

> In the family situation, however, the hypnotists (parents) are already hypnotized (by their parents) and are carrying out their instructions by bringing up their children in such a way, which includes not realizing that one is carrying out instructions: since one instruction is not to think that one is thus instructed. (Laing, 1973).

Rules Regarding the Recombining of Experience

Idiosyncratic patterns, or "rules of recombining", apply to the experience of each different ASC for each individual. The child abuser who cannot smile or apologize may be able to organize a bodily response typical of smiling, but within his or her normal state of consciousness. Associational rules prevent the recombining of experience that would make it possible to shift from a verbal misunderstanding to the display of a smile unless the typical stabilizing mechanism is used to increase comfort from within the typical ASC. The abuser may have no learned or understood way to go from social tension to smiling (and may give reasons why smiling cannot or ought not to be done).

SYMPTOM FORMATION AND ALTERED STATES

The inability to stabilize or the lack of alteration between appropriate states of consciousness creates stress. Moments of stress invite an overuse or misuse of the mechanisms and resources available in an ASC. The frequently stimulated or suppressed (unconscious) resources and patterns give rise to personal and social conflicts.

The development of symptoms in a family member often serves the function of evoking and stabilizing otherwise unstable resources among family members. In extremely rigid systems, the emergence of symptomatic behavior is a highly symbolic unconscious product of such "transpersonal collusion" (Laing, 1972).

Thus, we can examine individual and family systems in terms of ASC and recognize aspects that relate to Erickson's work with hypnosis and families. Erickson (1980) stated that to continue the process of inducing a trance should be regarded as a method of teaching patients a new manner of learning something, and thereby enabling them to discover unrealized capacities to learn, and to act in new ways.

This part of the chapter concludes in a fashion similar to the tales of yesteryear, in which the prince saves the girl, or today the girl gets the prince, or they both disappear together and are not heard from again.

THE CATASTROPHE

In ancient times, catastrophe, or the lysis, occurred naturally, that is, the fairy tale went as long as the storyteller kept talking or until teller or audience fell asleep or the story itself petered out.

In respect to Erickson, our modern tale will reiterate the four pillars of his work and leave the remainder to your imagination. Because of his naturalistic approach, his therapeutic work on the waking state was often indistinguishable from his work using hypnosis. Thus, the foundation of Erickson's work is the utilization of client behavior, indirect techniques, strategic therapy, and a naturalistic approach.

Erickson's approach made him an original in the history of hypnosis; his earlier motivation came from personal sources having to do with problems of learning and altered modes of sensory perceptual functioning rather than the traditional interests in psychopathology which was characteristic of earlier workers.

Basically, Erickson employs a heuristic, problem-solving procedure that may represent a new philosophical stance toward therapy and change (Haley, 1973). His uncommon therapy represents a departure from the logical practitioners, who see therapy only in terms of rectified personality theory.

Erickson took pleasure in demonstrating how psychological theories are limited by their own preconceived constructs. He would warn his students that hypothesis building based on <u>any</u> theory of personality can be a procrustean bed. His desire was to tailor the bed to fit the person, and he repeatedly teased the students by saying that he created a new theory for each client.

Erickson developed an approach referred to as utilization techniques. This approach combines acceptance and use of the client's ongoing behavior. It derives from an understanding that even behaviors that initially appear most resistive must be used to improve communication and motivation for therapy. Comprehending the client's states of experience, consciousness, and behavior are the foundations for utilization. Not to be confused with a client-centered approach, which passively accepts the client's experience, the utilization approach moves ahead to actively employ the current behavior or perception as a vehicle that helps therapy move to the next moment, the next stage, or the next goal.

Some practitioners believe that many people cannot be hypnotized (Spiegel, 1972). The utilization approach suggests that one not even need to be "relaxed" to be hypnotized. A compulsive floor pacer was asked, "Are you willing to cooperate with me by continuing to pace the floor, even as you are doing now?" "Willing?" he replied, "God, I've got to do it if I stay in the office." A 45 minute pattern of ever slowing instructions to guide the man's exact pacing around the office ensued. The verbal patter made increasing reference to the easy chair and the pleasure of resting in it. In this manner the client was able to use his apparent resistance as a step in the induction of a clinical state of hypnosis (Erickson, 1980). Thus the behavior that would be termed "resistance" was actually encouraged and used as a stepping stone to the next clinical goal.

Indirect suggestion is the last cornerstone of Erickson's hypnosis to be covered in this chapter. The pacing client was not told to sit in the chair and relax. Rather, Erickson chose his words in such a manner that the idea of being comfortably seated was allowed to arise from the client's own thinking. With the utilization approach, the client's customary "resistance" was bypassed because he was not directly told to do anything. Indirect suggestion provides only a gentle mental hint that focuses awareness, speaks in truisms, implies something, names possible alternatives, or speaks in purposefully general and vague terms. In this way, clients are free to form ideas with motivational aspects because these ideas are not alien and are not subjected to the same rule of censorship as are the apprehension and resistance present in the normal waking state.

Indirect suggestion is one of several indirect techniques. Others include anecdotes, stories that exchange ideas in a metaphoric form, and suggestions that are interspersed throughout other ostensible conversation. It is vital to recognize that the therapeutic use of indirect communication techniques does not make the clients have any particular experience or perception. Instead, clients are provided a type of stimulation that generally initiates the retrieval of novel experiences from another ASC or experience restricted by the "rules of recombining" that operate in the preferred ASC.

Repeated observations of this occurrence suggest that the subsystems of learned associations (commonly called the conscious mind) existing in the preferred ASC install most of the restrictions on experience. Indirect suggestion stimulates a search for unconscious process that is not censored in these consciously defended beliefs and conditioned perceptions. Thus, indirect suggestions, metaphor and anecdotes can tap therapeutic potentialities beyond the usual state of consciousness.

The remaining two foundations of Erickson's approach will be named but not discussed here. They are paradoxical symptom prescriptions and Ericksonian induction techniques.

A final note: a canon in the use of hypnosis is that one does not use it in areas where one would not be competent without the use of hypnosis. Meeting that principle, the induction of hypnosis is quickly learned; indeed, a hypnotic trance may be induced by reading instructions to a patient, and some practitioners have even resorted to having patients listen to induction on audiotapes. The induction of hypnosis is an art that skilled communication of ideas using cues from the subject to enhance and develop awareness and attention for the purpose of changing thoughts, feelings, and behavior.

When hypnosis is to be used during psychotherapy, it is helpful to prepare clients. Discuss with them their knowledge of hypnosis, clarify misconceptions, and instruct them as to what they may experience (i.e., "you will feel relaxed, attentive to my voice, calm"). Tell them what they can expect (the possibility that they will make some of the changes they wish to make in their lives). Some practitioners and especially academicians, used standardized tests of hypnotic susceptibility for the purpose of screening patients for hypnosis, while others (e.g., F. Weitzenhoffer, 1980) disagree with the use of such scales. The American Journal of Clinical Hypnosis, volume 21, issues 2 and 3, is devoted to discussions of hypnotic susceptibility scales. I generally do not use these scales in clinical practice. Most "motivated" people go into trance states easily, and most of the work that we do as psychotherapists does not require a state of hypnosis.

GLOSSARY

Catalepsy: Catalepsy refers to involuntary tonicity of the muscles (e.g., an arm may be placed in the air, the subject told that it is like an iron rod, and it may remain there still and rigid).

Deepening: Deepening is a reinduction procedure to allow the trance state to become more pronounced.

Depth of Trance: Depth of trance is loosely defined as the amount of relaxation and sensory alteration necessary to demonstrate various phenomena (e.g., partial amnesia, anesthesia, hallucinations).

Ideomotor Activity: Ideomotor activity refers to the capability of muscles to respond involuntarily to feelings, thoughts, and ideas; it is often used as a way of communicating with finger levitation when verbal communication tends to lighten the trance state. A variety of other trance and suggestion phenomena are found in W. Kroger's Clinical and Experimental Hypnosis, (1977).

Induction: Induction refers to the direction given to the client on how to achieve a hypnotic state, either in a verbal or nonverbal manner.

Trance: Synonymous with the word "hypnosis." The word "trance" seems to have a rather negative association for some people, perhaps because of stage hypnosis. I rarely use the term with a client. In fact, I may or may not use the word "hypnosis," although with one patient I failed to identify the procedure and she resented my using "hypnosis" without first getting her permission. It can be described in other terms, such as psychological relaxation.

PROFESSIONAL ORGANIZATIONS OFFERING WORKSHOPS AND TRAINING

The American Journal of Clinical Hypnosis
2250 East Devon Avenue, Suite 336
Des Plaines, IL, 60018

The American Society of Clinical Hypnosis
2250 East Devon Avenue, Suite 336
Des Plaines, IL, 60018

The International Journal of Clinical and Experimental Hypnosis, Subscription Sector
111 North 49th Street
Philadelphia, PA, 19139

The Society for Clinical and Experimental Hypnosis
128-A Kings Park Drive
Liverpool, NY, 13082

Steven Lankton Association
P.O. Box 958
Gulf Breeze, FL, 32561

REFERENCES

Berne, E. 1966. Principles of Group Treatment. New York: Grove.

Erickson, M. H. "Hypnotism." In E. L. Rossi, ed. The Collected Papers of Milton H. Erickson on Hypnosis. Vol. 3, Hypnosis Investigation of Psychodynamic Processes, pp. 21-26. New York: Irvington.

Erickson, M. H. 1980c. "Hypnotic Psychotherapy." In E. L. Rossi, ed. The Collected Papers of Milton H. Erickson on Hypnosis. Vol. 4, Innovative Hypnotherapy, pp. 35-38. New York: Irvington.

Erickson, M. H. 1980a. "Further Clinical Technique of Hypnosis: Utilization Techniques." In E. L. Rossi, ed. The Collected Papers of Milton H. Erickson on Hypnosis. Vol. 1, The Nature of Hypnosis and Suggestion, pp. 177-205. New York: Irvington.

Galvin, M., 1983. "Making Systematic Problem-Solving Work with Children." Journal of School Counseling, November.

Haley, J. 1973. Uncommon Therapy: The Psychiatry Techniques of Milton Erickson, M.D., New York: Ballantine.

Hartland, J. 1971. Medical and Dental Hypnosis. 2nd ed. Baltimore: Williams and Stratton.

Hilgard, E. R., and J. R. Hilgard. 1975. Hypnosis in the Relief of Pain, Los Altos, Calif.: William Kaufman.

Kroger, W. 1977. Clinical and Experimental Hypnosis. 2nd ed. Philadelphia: Lippincott. Laing, R. D. 1970. Knots. New York: Random House.

Laing, R. D. 1972. Politics of the Family and Other Essays. New York: Random House. 1972.

Lankton, S., and C. Lankton. 1983. The Answer Within: A Clinical Framework of Ericksonian Hypnotherapy. New York: Bruner/Mazel.

Mead, M. 1949. Male and Female: A Study of the Sexes in a Changing World. New York: Morrow.

Pearce, J. C. 1974. Exploring the Cracks in the Cosmic Egg. New York: Simon and Schuster.

Sheehan, P. W., and C. W. Perry. 1976. Methodologist of Hypnosis. Hillsdale, N.J.: Erlbaum.

Spiegel, H. 1972. "Eye Roll Test for Hypnotizabilty", American Journal of Clinical Hypnosis, 15: 25-28.

Tinterow, M. A. 1970. Foundations of Hypnosis: From Mesmer to Freud. Springfield, Ill. Charles C. Thomas.

Wolfberg, L. R. 1972. Hypnosis: Is It For You? New York: Harcourt Brace, Jovanich.

Zeig, J. K. 1980. A Teaching Seminar with Milton H. Erickson. New York: Bruner/Mazel.

PART III

NEW TRENDS IN RESEARCH IN PSYCHOTHERAPY

10

The Construction of a New Paradigm in Psychotherapy Research: An Urgent Need

Augusto Perez Gomez

In the following pages I will attempt to bring under scrutiny several concepts that, in my opinion, deserve a judicious examination in view of the impact of their current general acceptance. It was only during the last decade, and after some 40 years of activity in the field, that the pros and cons of traditional research methods began to be critically discussed. A few remarks, albeit cursory in their emphasis, had emerged in the literature, pointing out that such methods hardly could be adequately implemented, that the designs initially devised could almost never be conducted as planned, and that the data thereby gathered usually lacked clinical relevance. As a consequence, the endeavor ended. In most cases the authors neglected any continuation or further development of research in clinical practice. Adaptations to systematic research, on the other hand, signaled widespread chaos in the conceptual and theoretical bases of clinical practice. All sorts of contradictory data, speculations, theoretical analyses, ambiguous technical descriptions, and clusters of diagnostic categories overwhelmed the field, producing a state of confusion that prevented even a superficial examination. Given this state of affairs, it would be impossible to acknowledge any scientific status for psychotherapy.

In addition, a quarrel emerged over the crucial point of the problem to be studied: Is research in psychotherapy to investigate outcome or process? In previous papers I discussed this issue in some detail (Perez and Gomez, 1982; Perez et al., 1980). Suffice it to say that over the last two or more decades, several researchers have indicated the misleading effect of artificially separating these two questions of <u>what</u> changes are brought about and <u>how</u> they are produced. We cope with a big challenge, however, when we try to find a way to approach this problem in a comprehensive manner. That is, it is difficult to achieve well-ordered, exact knowledge for those who look for both ethics and "real" advances in application. Where, then, are we to find the optimal research model?

The experimental approach has been favored by the investigative tradition in general psychology and, in particular, psychotherapy. Even a casual look at scientific journals easily confirms this claim. My point is, however, that if a contrast is made between the amount of time, effort, people, and money invested in this type of research and their outcome in terms of the standards mentioned, then one must conclude that such investment lacks justification. Two main difficulties are to be considered, one of a practical nature, the other of a conceptual nature.

1. Experimental designs have a strict use of a number of procedures (precise evaluative criteria, clear construct formulation, unambiguous definitions, exact measurement and control of variables, comparison groups, etc.) that can seldom take place within the context of psychotherapy. I will address this issue later in this chapter.
2. Since the ultimate aim of an <u>experiment</u> lies beyond the uniqueness of subject and situation, its very purpose turns out to be the opposite of any given therapeutic endeavor. Every therapist has to adjust his or her behavior to the behavior of the subject, and this fact makes it virtually impossible to design experiments on the total therapeutic situation (although not so on selected parts of it). So, to the extent that the unforeseen essence of a therapeutic process has to be modified in order to adjust to some experimental methodology, the whole situation becomes artificial and, therefore, cannot be called "therapy" anymore. Also, the absence of adequate control procedures will not allow for the occurrence of "true" experiments, and data obtained this way will be, at best, ambiguous and open to many different, alternative explanations (Hyman and Berger, 1965).

The above ideas lead us to the core of our problem. There seems to be a notion, deeply rooted in Western thought, that no significant and valid knowledge can be produced without experimentation. However, the history of humankind provides us with many instances of the inadequacy of that notion (unless, of course, a circular type of reasoning is used by defining as "significant and valid" the knowledge that is produced by experimentation). Architecture lacks experimental foundation; so does art; so does astronomy (except for those aspects related to instrument construction); and so does history (as it is built today on the basis of precise documents). Most of the things we "know" about human behavior, sparse and equivocal, also lack this experimental foundation. All this does not necessarily mean that experimentation is incompatible with other types of knowledge; in fact, even art can be made through some sort of experiment. The point is that as forms of knowledge, all of them can survive with no experiments at all. With respect to their value, a variety of ways of knowing are dependent on the subject or object of study. Experiments provide the solution to some questions, but not to <u>all</u> questions.

It is easy to conclude that if a given method of study, even one highly valued in Western culture, involves such operations on the object to be studied, then the very problem disappears. Rather than accept this, we must question the method itself, instead of neglecting, ignoring, or devaluing the object. At this point, three issues only briefly mentioned above deserve some clarification.

First, a general proposition: It is possible to develop a psychotherapeutic science or, to be consistent with an earlier position (Perez et al., 1982), a discipline in search of "scientificity" without the practice of well structured, systematic, and solid research. The question is whether that research necessarily has to be objective in the experimental sense. Let us be reminded that objectivity is but some sort of intersubjective consensus (brilliantly defined by Carl R. Rogers in several publications) and that in objective form everything is touched by its sight. Perhaps this is one of the reasons why many clinicians reject current research models.

Second, a misunderstanding might occur if the ideas presented thus far were taken as a rejection of experimental methodology in the clinical field.

For years I have conducted experiments on schizophrenia (Perez, 1981a; Perez, Obregon, and Gomez, 1982; Perez, 1983). At least twice I investigated selected aspects of psychotherapy with experimental designs (Perez, Nur, and Suarez, 1981d; Perez, Bolanos, Cristo and Ramirez, 1982). My point is that experimental methods are totally insufficient to understand those phenomena that are of concern to the clinician, and that research should not be reduced only to problems amenable to experimental study.

Third, I would like to substantiate my opinion on the requirements of experimental designs. This opinion relates to the current development of our knowledge and, as such, does not imply any unmodifiable, general statement. The experimental model requires variable control and manipulation in order to convincingly show some relation between a number of procedures (described in clear terms, both conceptually and practically) and the outcome. In the psychotherapeutic realm this goal has many difficulties. I will mention only three.

1. Do we really know what the relevant variables are?

Usually, four are mentioned: therapist, subject, therapeutic style, and subject's environment. A casual examination shows that these are in fact "clusters" of variables. For an initial approach, it may be useful to deal with them as unitary factors, but we cannot overlook their extraordinary complexity and the multiplying effect of their interactions. We might run the risk of speaking of manipulation and control without actually knowing what is it that we control or manipulate. Systematic and coherent use of these methods might help in the analysis of concepts and in the refinement of techniques in analogous and nontherapeutic situations where common processes or events are already identified.

2. How do notions of manipulation and control function within the framework of therapeutic events?

In other words, how can these notions be implemented without altering the psychotherapeutic phenomenon itself? Even today, this question implies an unsolved problem for virtually all forms of therapy, including the simplest intervention schemes, when these are taken as integral situations rather than as mere opportunities for the application of specific, isolated techniques.

Since some therapists apparently think of psychotherapy as a "collection of techniques," it seems relevant to ask whether the clinician has to deal with problems or with people. If the answer is "problems," then my question may be ignored, because in these terms psychotherapy is not viewed as a relationship.

3. Can we really measure what takes place in the process? How can we discriminate the outcome of a therapeutic relationship from the results of a variety of factors and events unrelated to therapy? What are the criteria? Can we be certain that these criteria count at all? Are they valid? Are they value free? Most importantly, where do we find the measurement devices that supposedly outlive the critical charges of irrelevance or lack of testability?

To my knowledge there are no available answers to these questions.

If the goal is to attain a profound and realistic understanding of the events in the therapeutic situation, then experimentation does not appear to be the best avenue because of its remarkable limitation in both practical and conceptual terms. Nevertheless, parts of the therapeutic situation admit a judicious use of experimental approaches. For instance, some features, roles, or behavior of therapist and subject could be determined, as well as the nature and management of some intervention techniques or adequate and inadequate conditions for work. This brings forth my first proposal: It is imperative to discriminate between what can be analyzed via experimentation and what cannot. In my opinion, this essential step has not yet been taken.

The following suggestions do not deviate much from those offered by D. H. Ford and H. Urban (1967) as progressive differentiation of analytic strategies in accordance with the varying complexity of the problems under study.

A second possibility, useful for achieving valid and significant knowledge (although with limited generality), is the systematic use of single case studies. The case study has been the most favored method in our field, to the point of having been identified as <u>the</u> clinical method. Unfortunately, the failure here seems to be related to the "systematic" aspect. Modern technology allows us to gather very useful information and employ it in a wide variety of settings. (See Bolgar, 1965; Yates, 1970.) However, the number of studies in this category is small. We still have to cope with many methodological problems in the management, organization, and interpretation of data. The whole process may demand huge amounts of effort and time. Additionally, the tasks involved may be tedious, and generalization may not be as easily obtained as most researchers and theoreticians might require for scientific purposes. Case studies are initial and crucial steps in the development of an impartial cognitive science.

The third strategy, frequently used during the 1970s and not so much during the 1980s, is to use "analogue studies." These involve some degree of situational re-creation and permit manipulation, isolation, and quantitative scaling of variables that would not be possible in the real therapeutic scene. Regrettably, these procedures are not free from difficulties either. Given their "as if" nature, analogues imply a number of interpretive risks, mistakes, and abuses. Apparently this is the reason for the current mistrust. The proverbial pendulum in the history of psychology has swung from an enthusiastic defense of analogues to a massive rejection of them. In fact, many journals refuse analogue manuscripts submitted for publication and thus neglect their excellent information on technical aspects. Cautiously implemented, analogues are useful tools in hypothesis clarification and conceptual progress.

The works by K. I. Howard, D. E. Orlinsky, and their collaborators (K. I. Howard and D. E. Orlinsky, 1972; K. I. Howard, D. E. Orlinsky, and J. A. Hill, 1970; K. I. Howard, D. E. Orlinsky, and J. Perilstein, 1976; D. E. Orlinsky and K. I. Howard, 1978) represent a fourth possibility. These researchers, as well as some others, like D. J. Kiesler (1973) and T. Parson and E. Shils (1951), have developed a research model on the basis of participant observation. This model paves the way for evaluation of the subjective experience of both therapist and subject. Topics studied with this form of analysis range from "expectation evolution" to changes in the emotional process, perceptions on the relevance of the issues treated during a session, and development of consultation motives. The amount of data thus obtained is so great that the search for order and coherence presents a difficult task even with the aid of computers. On the other hand, anyone can see that a holistic view of a single therapeutic session (not to mention the entire process) will not emerge easily with this method. Although I have been able to refine several hypotheses relevant to my clinical practice (A. Perez, S. Gomez and M. Restrepo, 1980; instrument development; A. Perez and E. Vargas, 1981; expectation evolution; A. Perez and M. Torres, 1983; joint evolution of expectation and consultation motive), my optimism is rather low in view of the problems yet to be solved in areas such as design, data analysis, theoretical relevance, and practical implications of results.

On the basis of these ideas, it may be said that the area of research in psychotherapy might be compared to an unfinished puzzle. A great deal of talent on the part of those interested in advancing it will be needed to overcome the difficulties. The unexpected appearance of countless numbers of techniques and therapeutic styles has had a paradoxical effect, in that the need for integration in the theoretical, practical, and investigative spheres is more evident than ever before. Relevant instances of movement in this direction are those of Paul L. Wachtel (1977, 1983), Michael J. Mahoney (1981, 1982), Allen Ivey and Lynn Simek-Downing (1981), or Michel Legrand (1983). A clear trend is observed toward coincidence of interest, decrease of dogmatic stances, and search for a common language. The end product is not easily foreseen, but the endeavor is highly promising.

As psychotherapists, it is our duty to devote our energies to the search for new methodological conceptualizations, instead of forcing problems into their simplest forms with the purpose of handling them by means of strategies shown to be useful in other disciplines. Instead of deciding that problems are too complex and nothing can be done, a new approach to problem solving and new research designs may be necessary to cope adequately with this challenge. This is a most attractive opportunity because, hitherto, nobody has dared to meet it.

REFERENCES

Bergin, A. E. 1971. "The Evaluation of Therapeutic Outcomes." In A. E. Bergin and S. L. Garfield, eds. Handbook of Psychotherapy and Behavior Change: An Empirical Analysis. New York: Wiley.

Bergin, A. E., and M. J. Lambert. 1978. "The

Evaluation of Therapeutic Outcomes." In S. L. Garfield and A. E. Bergin eds. Handbook of Psychotherapy and Behavior Change. 2nd ed. New York: Wiley.

Bolgar, H. 1965. "The Case Study Method." In B. Wolman, ed. Handbook of Clinical Psychology. New York: McGraw-Hill, pp. 29-37.

Bordin, E. S. 1965. Research Strategies in Psychotherapies, New York: Wiley.

Corsini, R., ed. Handbook of Innovative Psychotherapies. New York: Wiley.

Ford, D. H., and H. Urban. 1967. "Psychotherapy." Annual Review of Psychology 18: 333-72.

Garfield, S. L. 1974. Clinical Psychology. The Study of Personality and Behavior. Chicago: Aldine.

Gottman, J., and H. Markman. 1978. "Experimental Designs in Psychotherapy Research." In S. L. Garfield and A. E. Bergin, eds. Handbook of Psychotherapy and Behavior Change. 2nd ed. New York: Wiley.

Howard, K. I., and D. E. Orlinsky. 1972. "Psychotherapeutic Process." In P. Mussen and M. Rosenzweig, eds. Annual Review of Psychology, 23.

Howard, K. I., and D. E. Orlinsky. 1986. "Process and Outcome in Psychotherapy." In S. L. Garfield and A. E. Bergin eds. Handbook of Psychotherapy and Behavior Change. 3d. ed. New York: Wiley, pp. 311-81.

Howard, K. I. 1970. D. E. Orlinsky and J. Hill, "Patients' satisfactions in psychotherapy as a function of patient-therapist pairing." Psychotherapy: Theory, Research and Practice, 7: 130-34.

Howard, K. I., Orlinsky, D. E., and J. Perilstein. 1976. "The contribution of therpists to patients' experiences in psychotherapy: A components of variance model for analyzing process data." Journal of Consulting and Clinical Psychology, 44: 520-26.

Hyman, R., and L. Berger. 1965. "The Effects of Psychotherapy: Discussion." International Journal of Psychiatry, 1: 317-22.

Ivey, A., and L. Simek-Downing. 1981. Counseling and Psychotherapy: Skills Theories and Practice. Englewood Cliffs, N.J.: Prentice-Hall.

Kiesler, D. J. 1973. The Process of Psychotherapy. Chicago: Aldine.

Lazarus, A., and G. Davidson. 1971. "Clinical Innovation in Research and Practice." In A. E.

Bergin, and S. L. Garfield, eds. Handbook of Psychotherapy and Behavior Change. New York: Wiley.

Legrand, M. 1983. "Terapias tradicionales y terapias modernas: diferencias y semejanzas." In A. Perez and F. Barrera, eds. Psicoterapieas 1983: Perspectivas de integracion. Bogotá: Uniandes.

Mahoney, M. J. 1981. "Clinical Psychology and Scientific Inquiry". International Journal of Psychology 16: 257-74.

Mahoney, M. J. 1982. "Psychotherapy and Human Change Processes." In Harve, J. H. and M. M. Parks, eds. The Master Lecture Series. Vol. 1., Psychotherapy Research and Behavior Change. Washington, D.C.: American Psychological Association.

Orlinsky, D. E., and K. I. Howard. 1978. "The Relation of Process to Outcome in Psychotherapy." In S. L. Garfield and A. E. Bergin, eds. Handbook of Psychotherapy and Behavior Change. 2nd ed. New York: Wiley.

Parson, T., and E. Shils, eds. Toward a General Theory of Action. Cambridge, Mass.: Harvard University Press.

Perez Gomez, A. n.d. "L'evaluation des effects des psicoterapias." Ph.D. diss. Louvain, Belgium: Catholic University.

Perez Gomez, A. 1981a. Psicoterapias: Enfoques teoricos, aplicados e investigativos. Bogotá: Uniandes.

Perez Gomez, A. 1983. "Pensamiento concreto-abstracto, dimension procesal reactiva y empleo del canal tactil en esquizofrenicos." Paper presented at the 14th Interamerican Congress of Psychology, Quito, Ecuador, July.

Perez Gomez, A., A. Bolanos, M. Cristo, and J. Ramirez. 1983. "Efecto de la terapia no directiva en ninos agresivos de clase socio-economica baja y alta." Unpublished manuscript. Bogotá: Universidad Javariana.

Perez Gomez, A., S. Gomez and M. Restrepo. 1980b. "Experiencia subjetiva en psicoterapia. Unpublished manuscript, Bogotá, Uniandes, 1980.

Perez Gomez, A., M. Nur, and Y. Suarez. 1981d. "Terapia de juego y adaptacion personal." In A. Perez Gomez, ed. Psicoterapias: enfoques teoricos aplicados e investigativos. Bogota: Uniandes, pp. 405-26.

Perez Gomez, A., P. Obregon, and E. Gomez. 1982. "Pensamiento concreto abstracto y dimension procesal-reactiva en esquizofrenicos."

Interamerican Journal of Psychology 15: 67-68.
Perez Gomez , A., and M. Torres. 1983. "Experiencia subjetiva en psicoterapia evolucion de expectativas en consultante y terapeuta." Unpublished manuscript. Bogotá: Uniandes.
Perez Gomez, A., and E. Vargas. 1981c. "Experiencia subjetiva en psicoterapia: Evolucion del motivo de consulta." Unpublished manuscript, Bogotá: Uniandes.
Runyan, W. 1982. "In Defense of the Case Study Method." American Journal of Orthopsychiatry. 52: 440-46.
Sargent, H. 1961. "Intrapsychic Changes: Methodological Problems in Psychotherapy Research." Psychiatry 24: 93-108.
Wachtel, P. L. 1977. Psychoanalysis and Behavior Therapy: Toward an Integration. New York: Basic Books.
Wachtel, P.L. 1983. "El significado social de las psicoterapias." In A. Perez Gomez and F. Barrera Currea, eds. Psicoterapias, 1983: perspectivas de integracion. Bogotá: Uniandes.
Yates, A. 1970. Behavior Therapy. New York: Wiley.

11

The Vanderbilt Psychotherapy Research Project: Past, Present, and Future

Hans H. Strupp

My early years as a psychotherapy researcher, around 1953, were marked by a special interest in the therapist's contribution to the treatment process. Based on clinical experience as well as the existing literature, I sensed intuitively that the person of the therapist had to play an important part in the therapeutic process, determining its quality and outcome. I never went so far as Carl R. Rogers (1957), however, who declared that the "therapist offered conditions" of warmth, empathy, genuineness, and unconditional positive regard that were the "necessary and sufficient conditions." As my experience grew and as I began to carry out a series of analogue studies (H. Strupp, 1960), I came to believe even more firmly that any meaningful definition of psychotherapy would have to accommodate personal qualities of the therapist that are brought to bear on the therapeutic interaction with a given patient. Thus, to describe psychotherapy in terms of its theoretical orientation or techniques, as was common then and still is now, provides a truncated view of what is essentially a complex human relationship in a specialized context. By this reasoning, what the therapist communicates by attitudes, gestures, and innuendo must be studied and understood as carefully as the techniques he or she uses. Briefly, psychotherapy is never adequately defined as a "treatment modality" or as set of "technical procedures." This position has important implications for how one conceptualizes psychotherapy as a "health care technology" and also calls into question the "clinical trials" approach to research. Progress has been made in studying the nature of the therapeutic influence, the primary task of research, but we have a long way to go in capturing the elusive qualities of what is therapeutic, antitherapeutic, or simply inert.

My early research, limited as it was in terms of resources, access to process and outcome data, and available technology, made a beginning contribution to the documentation of important differences among therapists and led to methodological advances in assessing the therapist's contribution (H. Strupp, 1957). In short, we began to differentiate between "technical" (specific) and "nontechnical" (nonspecific) factors, the latter referring to the therapist's human qualities that subtly, but decisively, suffused and were integrally related to his or her techniques. Others, notably Jerome Frank (J. Frank, 1973) were pursuing similar conceptualizations and inquiries. Basically, however, as we concluded later, this way of looking at the therapist's contributions has serious pragmatic limitations and inherent conceptual flaws (S. F. Butler and H. Strupp, 1986; W. P. Henry, 1958). For research purposes, scales may be developed to demonstrate that a given therapist is "adhering" to the technical dictates of a particular theoretical orientation to psychotherapy. These technical interventions occur, however, in the context of a multifaceted, ever changing human relationship between patient and therapist. The ultimate therapeutic impact of a therapist's intervention results from the <u>meaning</u> of the exchange to the patient, and "meaning" cannot be divided into "specific" and "nonspecific" factors. Therefore, lest we be caught up in an unfortunate reification, I now feel that we should abandon or reformulate the problem.

VANDERBILT I

What came to be known as the Vanderbilt Psychotherapy Project, or more specifically the Vanderbilt I Study, "Specific vs. Nonspecific Factors in Psychotherapy: A Controlled Study of Outcome" (H. Strupp and S. Hadley, 1979), began following collaboration with Allen E. Bergin which extended over a period of several years, beginning in the late 1960s, and culminated in <u>Changing Frontiers in the Science of Psychotherapy</u> (A. Bergin and H. Strupp, 1972). We were commissioned by the NIMH to explore whether large-scale collaborative studies were feasible. We concluded that the time was not ripe for such studies, but we did gain a better understanding of areas in which significant advances might be made. In the early 1970s, after several years of pilot work, the Vanderbilt I Study was initiated and lasted almost ten years.

Using a no treatment control group design, the Vanderbilt group sought to explore the incremental effects of therapist training on process and outcome via the then dominant paradigm of "specific" and "nonspecific" factors. Using a reasonably specific patient population (in this case, male college students suffering from moderately severe anxiety, depression, and social withdrawal), we compared the outcomes of patients treated by college professors selected for their understanding and warmth (thought to represent in relatively pure form the nonspecific factors believed common to all psychotherapies) with patients treated by experienced professional therapists. It was hypothesized that systematic differences in outcome favoring professional therapists would constitute evidence for the unique importance of technical factors. The therapy was time-limited (up to 25 hours), and techniques were allowed to vary freely. The professional therapists who had no special expertise in time-limited therapy were either psychoanalytic or client-centered/humanistic in their theoretical orientation.

The major results of the study, together with its unintended extrapolations to professional training and contemporary political trends, are well known. We replicated the common finding that some form of psychotherapy is better than no treatment, but it seemed to make little difference who administered it. In retrospect, neither the conceptualization nor the experimental design were felicitous. We learned a painful and important lesson regarding the extent to which enduring and potentially faulty blanket conclusions may be reached on the basis of group mean analyses. Had we stopped with the traditional group comparisons we would have been left with very little, aside from the distressing and, as we later discovered, inaccurate conclusion that professional training contributes little to positive therapeutic outcomes.

Fortunately, in contrast with most studies previously undertaken, we had made careful assessments from multiple perspectives: patient, therapist, and evaluating clinician (H. Strupp and S. Hadley, 1977). Most important, we had complete sound recordings of every therapy hour and videotapes of selected ones. We were also blessed with several generations of unusually gifted, creative graduate students and postdoctoral fellows. Finally, the continuing confidence and support of NIMH proved indispensable. With this auspicious constellation of factors, we carried out a sizable number of studies that explored in detail and depth the vagaries and vicissitudes of the patient-therapist interaction in individual cases. Comparisons between clients with high and low levels of change seen by the same therapist were particularly fruitful. To aid these explorations we developed several new methodological tools, notably the Vanderbilt Psychotherapy Process Scale (VPPS) and the "Vanderbilt Negative Indicators Scale (VNIS) (Suh, et al., 1986), which were used in assessing salient aspects of the therapists' and patients' behaviors as well as their interaction. By deliberately alternating between the quantitative measures and the clinical data, we sought to advance our understanding of both. The lessons we learned were built into the Vanderbilt II Study, to be described shortly.

Research Results

Result No. 1.

Neither professional therapists nor college professors were notably effective in treating patients with more characterological problems, such as pronounced hostility, pervasive mistrust, negativism, inflexibility, and antisocial or asocial tendencies. The suitability of these patients for time-limited therapy emerged as questionable in our retrospective assessments. On the other hand, the group data had obscured the finding that professional therapists had often been more effective than lay therapists with patients showing the following characteristics: high motivation for psychotherapy; ability to form a good therapeutic relationship (working alliance) early in treatment; and relative absence of long-standing maladaptive patterns of relating to significant others.

The foregoing is not meant to imply that professional therapists were most effective with the least disturbed patients. Rather, these therapists were particularly effective with patients whose personality resources and capacity for collaboration allowed them to take maximal advantage of the kind of relationship and traditional techniques preferred by the therapist. These findings are in general agreement with the literature (Kernberg et al.,

1972).

Result No. 2.

The quality of the therapeutic relationship seemed to be established quite early in therapy and proved to be an important predictor of outcome in this time-limited context. In particular, the therapy tended to be successful if by the third session the patient felt accepted, understood, and liked by his therapist (G. J. Waterhouse, 1979). Conversely, premature termination or failure tended to result if these conditions were not met early in treatment. In addition, we obtained preliminary evidence that reasonably accurate predictions of process and outcome can be made from the initial session, specifically in terms of judgments relating to the patient's motivation for therapy (L. J. Keithly et al., 1980). Most important, we found no evidence that an initially negative or highly ambivalent patient-therapist relationship was significantly modified in the course of therapy under study, and the patients' perceptions of the therapeutic relationship were found to remain fairly stable throughout therapy and to the follow-up period.

Result No. 3.

The quality of the therapeutic relationship appeared to depend heavily on the patient's ability to relate comfortably and productively to the therapist in the context of a traditional therapeutic framework. This capacity, in turn, seemed to be a function of the patient's personality resources and suitability for time-limited therapy. (See result no. 1.) In short, there was compelling evidence that the quality of the patient-therapist relationship was significantly, although not entirely, determined by patient variables.

Result No. 4.

Professional therapists gave little evidence of adapting their therapeutic approaches or techniques to the specific characteristics and needs of individual patients. Instead, the kind of relationship they offered and the techniques they employed were relatively invariant. Similarly, therapists did not tailor their techniques in specific ways to the resolution of "target symptoms," nor did they seem to formulate specific therapeutic goals of their own that were then systematically pursued in therapy.

Result No. 5.

Professional psychotherapists, in general, had little success in confronting or resolving the marked negative reactions characteristic of the more difficult patients. Instead, they tended to react negatively and counter-therapeutically to a patient's hostility, mistrust, inflexibility, and pervasive resistances, thereby perhaps reinforcing the patient's poor self-image and related difficulties. The results of such interactions tended to be negative attitudes on the part of the patient toward the therapist and the therapy; premature termination; and/or a poor therapeutic outcome (no change or negative change). For detailed analyses, see my three articles in volume 37 of the Archives of General Psychiatry (Strupp, 1980a, 1980b, 1980c).

These results have significant implications for research and clinical practice.

Patient Selection

Patients with substantial personality resources, high levels of motivation for therapy, relatively circumscribed problems, and the capacity to work productively within a traditional therapeutic framework are likely to show the greatest and most rapid improvement. From the therapist's standpoint, these persons usually are the most desirable and rewarding patients. When viewed from the broader perspective of the needs of society and the future development of psychotherapy, however, these are the least problematic cases.

By contrast, patients falling short of optimal suitability for short-term approaches (according to the criteria mentioned above) represented by far the largest segment of the patient population. Paradoxically, while these individuals are in the greatest need of professional services, they are also the ones who have been most neglected by mental health professional. This judgment applies with particular force to short-term dynamic psychotherapy, which has traditionally focused on the selection and treatment of the most promising candidates (Koss and Butcher, 1986). It is noteworthy in this regard that the extensive contemporary literature dealing with borderline conditions and narcissistic personality disorders is almost entirely devoted to long-term intensive therapy, (e.g., Kernberg, 1975; Kohut, 1971).

Conclusion 1.

In order for psychotherapy to more adequately meet the needs of patients as well as society, it is essential to focus attention upon patients who have been rejected as suitable candidates for short-term psychotherapy and to explore systematically the extent to which such patients can be treated more effectively by a well defined, time-limited approach.

Patient Assessment

Considering the complexity of the human personality, it is perhaps not surprising that even when assessment procedures are designed to select a homogeneous group of patients, the resulting samples are likely to include individuals who differ widely on a number of dimensions considered critical to their suitability for time-limited psychotherapy. For example, the initial patient selection was based on a significant elevation ($T > 60$) of scales 2 (depression), 7 (psychoasthenia), and 0 (social introversion) of the Minnesota Multiphasic Personality Inventory. Although we did not insist that all patients be "pure" 2-7-0's, marked variability was observed in the subsample that met this criterion. These patients showed wide variations in terms of character structure, ranging from mild neurotic disturbances in a relatively well functioning personality organization to severe obsessionals, character disorders, and even a few borderline conditions. Thus the term "homogenous," when applied in the research literature, is likely to be quite relative, even under controlled conditions.

In the light of our findings and those of others (Davanloo, 1978, 1980; Malan, 1976, 1979; Sifneos, 1972, 1979), additional criteria of significance for treatment planning should include: (1) severity of characterological disturbances (negativism, pervasive mistrust, and rigidity), (2) degree of impairment in coping ability, (3) quality of past interpersonal relationships, (4) motivation for change, and (5) presence of "core conflictual themes" (L. Luborsky, 1977) or central issues that allow for the establishment of a dynamic focus. Despite the importance of these qualities to the determination of a patient's suitability for a particular treatment approach, such careful assessments are typically not made in clinical practice. C. W. McLemore and L. S. Benjamin (1979) present a strong argument that traditional nosology, instead of focusing on <u>interpersonal behavior</u> (the proper focus for planning and executing psychotherapy), employs categories that, in the view of numerous authors (e.g., R. C. Carson, 1969, p. 224) are "largely meaningless."

<u>Conclusion 2.</u>

Psychiatric assessments must be sharpened to include: (1) evaluations of the patient's interpersonal functioning; (2) determinations of the patient's suitability for time-limited psychotherapy in terms of the criteria that have been identified as important prognostic indicators; and (3) reformulation of the patient's presenting complaints in terms of central issues or themes that lend themselves to focused therapeutic interventions. In order to effect more specific treatment planning, these determinations must become an integral part of the assessment process. Through this step, a closer link will be forged between diagnosis, formulation of therapeutic goals, techniques, and outcomes.

Therapeutic Operations

As shown by our analyses of patient-therapist interactions, professional therapists tended to use a broad-gauged approach aimed at helping patients achieve insight into certain aspects of their current difficulties. Although the treatment was time-limited, the psychodynamic therapists typically followed the analytic model of long-term intensive psychotherapy. Accordingly, they adopted a passive-expectant stance, left the initiative for introducing topics to the patient, and largely confined their activity to clarifications and interpretations of conflictual patterns. These therapists tended to provide relatively little warmth and support, did not focus on the specific problems identified at the beginning of treatment, rarely acquainted the patients with the nature of the therapeutic process, and infrequently confronted the patients' negative personal reactions. To summarize, the therapists' approach tended to be relatively invariant, and their patients were expected to feel comfortable with and respond favorably to the requirements of this therapeutic framework without significant efforts on the therapist's part.[1] It should be noted that this approach reflects the model followed in many training centers for psychologists and psychiatrists, despite the fact that the majority of patients are unable to take optimal advantage of this regimen. Furthermore, as shown by our research results, the absence of a good "fit" between pertinent patient characteristics and the therapist's framework frequently led to an impasse early in treatment, such as a poor therapeutic alliance, premature termination, or a poor outcome.

Of particular significance to the course and outcome of treatment were therapists' negative personal reactions to patients whose resistance took the form of anger, hostility, negativism, and pervasive mistrust. These negative reactions apparently were often outside of the therapists' awareness and occurred despite adequate theoretical understanding of counter-transference. In view of these findings, we believe that systematic efforts must be made to help therapists deal with this problem.

Conclusion 3.

To realize the full potential for short-term dynamic psychotherapy, therapists should receive specialized training, with particular emphasis on the following elements:

1. Techniques should be geared optimally to the achievement of reasonably specific therapeutic objectives identified early in the course of treatment. Crucial here is the isolation of a central issue, dynamic focus, or "theme."
2. The therapeutic process should be designed to meet the unique needs of the individual patient, as opposed to the tacit assumption that the patient conform to the therapist's notion of an "ideal" therapeutic framework. Techniques should be applied flexibly, sensitively, and in ways maximally meaningful to the patient.
3. Steps should be taken to foster a good therapeutic relationship (working alliance) from the beginning of therapy, thus enhancing the patient's active participation and creating a sense of collaboration and partnership.
4. Negative transference reactions should be actively confronted and worked through at the earliest therapeutically propitious time.
5. Concerted efforts should be made to help therapists recognize and deal with negative personal reactions, which are characteristically engendered by patients manifesting hostility, anger, negativism, rigidity, and similar resistances.

6. While time-limited psychotherapy poses particular challenges to all therapists (especially demands for greater activity and directiveness), they should resist temptations to persuade the patient to accept a particular "solution," impose their values, and in other respects diminish the patient's strivings for freedom and autonomy.
7. Rather than viewing psychotherapy predominantly as a set of "technical operations" applied in a vacuum, therapists must be sensitive to the importance of the human elements in all therapeutic encounters. In other words, unless the therapist takes an interest in the patient as a person and succeeds in communicating this interest and commitment, psychotherapy becomes a caricature of a good human relationship.
8. Closely related to the foregoing, therapists should keep in mind that all good therapeutic experiences lead to increments in the patient's self-acceptance and self-respect. Consequently, constant care must be taken to promote such experiences and to guard against interventions that might have opposite effects.

The foregoing terse summary does scant justice to the empirical bases of our inferences, conclusions, and recommendations. The best we can do is to refer the interested reader to the body of articles, chapters, dissertations, and manuals that undergird our assertions.

VANDERBILT II

Following completion of the basic Vanderbilt I analyses, a three-year period of developmental work was undertaken, during which time we attempted to translate the knowledge distilled from these analyses into a major new research project. We had discovered the crucial importance of a good working alliance and the speed with which the quality of the alliance seemed to be formed. We had also uncovered a glaring need for specialized training of therapists to enable them to bring greater focus to short-term therapy and to more quickly recognize and ameliorate potential counter-transference reactions with difficult individuals. If these goals were accomplished, we believed that it would be possible to extend the range of patients normally deemed suitable for short-term interventions, thus fulfilling an important public health need.

A number of research issues also had to be addressed. We had grown disenchanted with the clinical trials, or "horse race," approach to research and had abandoned the specific-nonspecific dichotomy as well. As noted earlier, we had also become critical of traditional forms of psychiatric assessment and diagnosis. In short, we had come to view the interpersonal dimension as central to understanding the nature of psychotherapy and, hence, increasingly focused on studying the interpersonal process between patient and therapist.

In keeping with these lines of reasoning, rather than being a traditional outcome study, the Vanderbilt II investigation focused on intensive exploration of the patient-therapist relationship, with emphasis on the manner in which specialized training might improve the quality of the therapeutic relationship, especially with difficult patients. To this end, pilot work included the development and field testing of a manual and adherence scale for Time-Limited Dynamic Psychotherapy (TLDP; Strupp and Binder, 1984). The TLDP manual is based on psychodynamic and interpersonal principles as adapted specifically to the demands of short-term treatment. The procedures are detailed for establishing a "dynamic focus" (a central cyclical maladaptive interpersonal pattern), the working through of which becomes the goal of therapy. To accomplish this goal, TLDP places its chief emphasis on the close scrutiny, understanding, and management of ongoing interpersonal transactions in the therapeutic relationship and a structured approach to time limits and termination.[2] Thus, while TLDP is founded upon and consistent with traditional analytic approaches to therapy, it calls for greater activity by the therapist and emphasizes observable interpersonal behaviors over more abstract concepts relating to defensive and intrapsychic structure.

In planning a new project, our research strategies and methodologies had to accomodate this conceptualization of psychotherapy as an exquisitely interpersonal endeavor, as opposed to a set of techniques administered mechanically to modify impersonal "symptoms." We had noted in Vanderbilt I that traditional assessment procedures often failed to directly address patient characteristics that facilitate or impede a patient's entry into a good working alliance with the therapist. In an attempt to overcome this problem, we developed the Capacity for Dynamic Process Scale (CDPS, Thackrey et al., 1985) which was designed to assess a patient's relative suitability for TLDP and was used to place incoming patients along a continuum of relative "difficulty." In conjunction with the CDPS, we developed a specialized, semi-structured interview aimed at identifying salient, problematic interpersonal patterns, as well as providing a behavioral measure of the patient's performance in a situation similar to therapy.

Finally, as we have implied, we viewed the patient's presenting difficulties as integrally related to the perpetuation of maladaptive patterns of interpersonal behavior, patterns that tend to be reenacted with the therapist. Thus, from a research standpoint, we needed to find better ways to capture the intricacies of the dynamic interactions in the therapeutic dyad. Historically, circumflex models have provided the most theoretically cogent and psychometrically sound method of measuring interpersonal behaviors (cf. Wiggins, 1982, for a review). From the available models, we chose to use the Structural Analysis of Social Behavior (SASB: L. S. Benjamin, 1974, 1982), as we felt it represented the most sophisticated and clinically relevant system for measuring both interpersonal process and therapeutic content. SASB permits an extremely fine grained analysis of virtually any interpersonal event and uses small rating units requiring relatively low levels of inference while permitting high levels of specificity. The addition of SASB based Intrex questionnaires enabled us to chart, in a common metric, the patient's presenting interpersonal symptomatology, the dyadic interpersonal process of therapy, and changes in intrapsychic structure and ongoing relationships. This allows research data to follow the principle of problem-treatment-outcome (PTP) congruence (Schacht et al., in press), a principle we feel is vital to making maximum conceptual sense from research results.

The Vanderbilt II protocol was structured so that each participating therapist served as his or her own control, avoiding what we felt to be less productive experimental designs based on a clinical trials approach. Sixteen experienced therapists (eight clinical psychologists and eight psychiatrists, each with a minimum of three years' post-residency or post-internship experience) treated two patients before and two patients after six months of specialized TLDP training during which time they saw an additional supervised case. The 80 project patients were broadly representative of an adult outpatient sample and were seen for a maximum of 25 sessions. Multiple measures of initial patient status, therapy process, adherence to TLDP principles, and outcome were obtained from the perspectives of patients, therapists, and independent evaluators as appropriate.

In its most basic form, Vanderbilt II was a study of the effects of a specific training procedure. As such, three main hypotheses were addressed: (1) TLDP is a set of specifiable principles and techniques that can be taught to experienced clinicians and that will influence the manner in which these therapists conduct psychotherapeutic treatment; (2) therapy conducted along TLDP guidelines will result in improved process and outcome; and (3) because TLDP specifically addresses the problem of interpersonal difficulties in the therapeutic relationship, the greatest relative improvements in process and outcome will occur with patients whose potential for effective participation in short-term dynamic therapy is considered relatively low. As of this writing, full-scale analyses of the Vanderbilt II data have just begun, and thus we cannot definitively answer the foregoing hypotheses. However, our experience over the course of the project has led us to some tentative conclusions and has already pointed toward our future research efforts.

As might be anticipated, the results of such a large scale, multi-faceted project are complex and thus difficult to summarize. One major finding of immediate importance to the field, however, involves the limits of "manualization," that is, the belief that one has adequately and precisely specified the "treatment variable" through the use of manualized training procedures and objective independent ratings of "adherence." As a group, the research therapists clearly learned to verbalize and apply TLDP principles to the extent necessary to meet adequate technical adherence standards. However, the patterns of skill acquisition appear to be complex, with varying patient characteristics adding additional complexity to the findings. Interpersonal processes may differ dramatically in cases of similar levels of technical adherence. We have also come to believe that it may be more difficult than originally believed to judge the suitability of patients for short-term dynamic therapy, at least as based on a single interview by an independent clinician. Finally, we have experienced frustration with the relatively crude state of the art of outcome measurement devices.

While the pursuit of a single, unambiguous indicator of "outcome" is undoubtedly fruitless, we feel that important advances can and should be made in the conceptualization and measurement of therapeutic change.

THE FUTURE OF THE VANDERBILT PROJECT

It is perhaps comforting, in an ironic way, that after a 35-year span that saw shifting research conceptualizations, a myriad of important and sometimes disturbing findings, and significant advances in research technology, we continue to confirm the initial intuitive belief in the importance of the person of the therapist. In the last few years we have begun to understand more about the therapist's early life experiences and the manner in which the therapist's own intrapsychic structure can color the interpersonal transactions in therapy that seem to be such crucial mediators of positive therapeutic outcome (W. P. Henry et al., 1986; W. P. Henry, 1986; J. C. Christenson et al., 1987). Conversely, we have also published research findings emphasizing the primary importance of pre-existing patient characteristics (Comparison 4, Strupp, 1980). Indeed, we now feel that both positions are correct if the therapeutic process is viewed as a momentary dyadic state, and not a quantative collection of unilateral acts.

This deceptively simple viewpoint has important implications for our continued exploration of more effective therapist training procedures. By this we mean that the interpersonal modes of action (which create momentary dyadic process states) with which technical prescriptions are carried out need to be more directly addressed in training. The type of fundamental interpersonal perceptual and action skills training we envision differs dramatically from traditional modes of therapeutic training. We will continue to seek improved methods for making therapists not only more aware of ongoing interpersonal transactions, but also able to direct them within the basic TLDP approach.

In place of large scale, quasi-experimental designs, we envision a more flexible research structure. This structure would permit, through a prospective research design, the processes of description, explanation, and prediction to evolve recursively, by using retrospective analyses of the large existing Vanderbilt II data set to direct ongoing therapies. While we will continue to use group analyses to uncover patterns and trends, we increasingly believe that intensive single case studies of exemplars of these patterns are required in order to achieve a fuller understanding of complex clinical phenomena. In this regard, two guiding principles for future analyses seem important. The first principle is to search for patterns across a number of concurrently measured process and outcome instruments, thus achieving a greater contextual validity for any single measure (see Greenberg, 1986, for a more complete discussion). The second principle involves an attempt to develop a structured, instrument-guided approach to case study that will permit aggregation and replication across cases. Finally, we will continue the difficult task of developing improved procedures and instruments for measuring the process and outcome of therapy.

In conclusion, let us state our conviction that the field of psychotherapy research remains in an embryonic state. To some, the collected wisdom based on research generated by the field adds up to a small number of general conclusions, such as "some form of therapy seems superior to no therapy for the majority of patients, but the 'type' of therapy seems to have little effect." On the other hand, we are now able to chart, in a fine grained manner, subtle interpersonal nuances that appear to have profound effects on the overall efficacy of individual therapies. When one steps back from such dichotomies, however, it is clear that important advances have occurred. In the 1950s it was considered controversial to even ask therapists to make hypothetical responses to therapeutic situations. At that time, the "black box" of the therapist's office was sacred and unquestioned, while now we routinely videotape therapeutic sessions. Over the history of the Vanderbilt psychotherapy research and practice, we have investigated many aspects of the psychotherapeutic practices, and we have done so through the pursuit of a better understanding of the therapeutic process. In the future, we hope to pursue this path by incorporating insights from research into studies of improved therapist training methods. Perhaps the time is not far off when practicing clinicians will be able to make use of the insights gained by researchers, thus consummating a partnership that has been slow in developing.

NOTES

1. While it was true that the therapists' overall technical stance varied little from patient to patient, later analyses (W. P. Henry et al., 1986) revealed subtle but extremely important differences in the interpersonal transactional processes the same therapist enacted with different patients.

2. Although for practical and strategic reasons we work with time-limited therapies, we believe that this model is equally compatible with therapies of no longer duration. J. L. Binder, W. P. Henry, and I (1987) outlined our views on the efficacy of bringing a short-term approach to long-term therapy.

REFERENCES

Benjamin, L. S. 1974. "Structural Analysis of Social Behavior." Psychological Review 81: 392-425.

Benjamin, L. S. 1982. "Use of Structural Analysis of Social Behavior to Guide Intervention in Therapy." In J. C. Anchin and D. J. Kiesler, eds. Handbook of Interpersonal Psychotherapy. New York: Pergamon.

Bergin, A. E. and H. H. Strupp, eds. 1972. Changing Frontiers in the Science of Psychotherapy. Chicago: Aldine-Atherton.

Butler, S. F. & H. H. Strupp. 1986. "Specific and Nonspecific Factors in Psychotherapy: A Problematic Paradigm for Psychotherapy Research." Psychotherapy 23, no. 1: 30-40.

Carson, R. C. 1969. Interaction Concepts of Personality. Chicago: Aldine.

Christenson, J. C., T. W. Lane, and H. H. Strupp, Pre-Therapy Interpersonal Relations and Introject as Reflected in the Therapeutic Process. Presented to the Society for Psychotherapy Research (SPR), Ulm, FRG.

Davanloo, H. 1978. Basic Principles and Techniques in Short-Term Dynamic Psychotherapy. New York: Spectrum.

Davanloo, H., ed. 1980. Short-Term Dynamic Psychotherapy. New York: Jason Aronson.

Frank, J. D. 1973. Persuasion and Healing: A Comparartive Study of Psychotherapy. Baltimore: Johns Hopkins University Press.

Greenberg, L. S. 1986. "Research Strategies." In L. S. Greenberg W. M. Pinsoff, eds. The

Psychotherapeutic Process: A Research Handbook. New York: Guilford Press.
Henry, W. P. 1958. "The Time Released Placebo: A Reply to Critelli and Neuman." American Psychologist 40: 289.
Henry, W. P. 1986. "Interpersonal Process in Psychotherapy." Dissertation.
Henry, W. P., T. E. Schacht, and H. H. Strupp. 1986. "Structural analysis of Social Behavior: Application to a Study of Interpersonal Process in Differential Psychotherapeutic Outcome." Journal of Consulting and Clinical Psychology 54, no. 1: 27-31.
Keithly, L. J., S. J. Samples, and H. H. Strupp. 1980. "Patient Motivation as a Predictor of Process and Outcome in Psychotherapy." Psychotherapy and Psychosomatics 33: 87-97.
Kernberg, O. F., E. D. Burstein, L. Coyne, A. Appelbaum, L. Horwitz, and H. Voth. 1972. "Psychotherapy and Psychoanalysis: Final Report of the Menninger Foundation's Psychotherapy Research Project." Bulletin of the Menninger Clinic 36, 1-275.
Kernberg, O. F. 1975. Borderline Conditions and Pathological Narcissism. New York: Jason Aronson.
Kohut, H. 1971. The Analysis of the Self. New York: International Universities Press.
Koss, M. P. and J. N. Butcher. 1986. "Research on Brief Psychotherapy." In S. L. Garfield, and A. E. Bergin, eds. 3rd ed. Handbook of Psychotherapy and Behavior Change. New York: Wiley, pp. 627-70.
Luborsky, L. 1977. "Measuring a Pervasive Psychic Structure in Psychotherapy: The Core Conflictual Relationship Theme." In N. Freedman, and S. Grand, eds. Communicative Structures and Psychic Structures. New York: Plenum, pp. 367-95.
Malan, D. H. 1976. The Frontier of Brief Psychotherapy: An Example of the Convergence of Research and Clinical Practice. New York: Plenum.
McLemore, C. W. and L. S. Benjamin. 1979. "Whatever Happened to Interpersonal Diagnosis?" American Psychologist 34: 17-34.
Rogers, C. R. 1957. "The Necessary and Sufficient Conditions of Therapeutic Personality Change." Journal of Consulting Psychology 22: 95-103.
Schacht, T. E., H. H. Strupp, and W. P. Henry. In press. Problem-Treatment-Outcome Congruence: A Principle Whose Time Has Come.

Sifneos, P. W. 1972. Short-Term Psychotherapy and Emotional Crisis. Cambridge, Mass.: Harvard University Press.

Sifneos, P. E. 1979. Short-Term Dynamic Psychotherapy: Evaluation and Technique. New York: Plenum Press.

Strupp, H. H. 1957. "A Multidimensional System for Analyzing Psychotherapeutic Techniques." Psychiatry 20: 293-306.

Strupp, H. H. 1960. Psychotherapists in Action: Explorations of the Therapist's Contribution to the Treatment Process. New York: Grune and Stratton.

Strupp, H. H. 1980a. "Success and Failure in Time-Limited Psychotherapy: A Systematic Comparison of Two Cases." (Comparison 1.) Archives of General Psychiatry 37: 595-603.

Strupp, H. H. 1980b. "Success and Failure in Time-Limited Psychotherapy: A Systematic Comparison of Two Cases." (Comparison 2.) Archives of General Psychiatry 37: 708-16.

Strupp, H. H. 1980c. "Success and Failure in Time-Limited Psychotherapy: With Special Reference to the Performance of a Lay Counselor." (Comparison 3.) Archives of General Psychiatry 37: 831-41.

Strupp, H. H. and J. L. Binder. 1984. Psychotherapy in a New Key: A Guide to Time-Limited Dynamic Psychotherapy. New York: Basic Books.

Strupp, H. H. and S. Hadley. 1979. "A Tripartite Model of Mental Health and Therapeutic Outcomes." American Psychologist 32: 187-96.

Suh, C. S., S. S. O'Malley, and H. H. Strupp. 1986. "The Vanderbilt Process Measures: The Psychotherapy Process Scale (VPPS) and the Negative Indicators Scales (VNIS)." In L. S. Greenberg and W. M. Pinsoff, eds. The Psychotherapeutic Process: A Research Handbook. New York: Guilford.

Thackrey, M., S. F. Butler, and H. H. Strupp. 1985. "Measurement of Patient Capacity for Dynamic Process." Paper presented to the Society for Psychotherapy Research, Evanston, Illinois, June.

Waterhouse, G. J. 1979. "Perceptions of Facilitative Therapeutic Conditions as Predictors of Outcome in Brief Therapy." Paper presented at the European conference of the Society for Psychotherapy Research, Oxford, England.

Wiggins, J. S. 1982. "Circumflex Models of

Interpersonal Behavior in Clinical Psychology." In P. C. Kendall and J. N. Butcher, eds. Handbook of Research Methods in Clinical Psychology. New York: Wiley.

12

Myths, Realities, and Alternatives to Clinical Trials

Edward S. Bordin

For my review of research and evaluation in psychotherapy I chose as a point of departure the examination of the clinical trial. Research in psychotherapy is entering into a new phase, and for the moment, developments have focused attention on the clinical trial as the medium through which these new approaches will be demonstrated. In the United States, the National Institute of Mental Health collaborative study of alternative treatments of depression has captured the center of attention. The mere size of this project, involving many clinical facilities and extremely large expenditures of funds, attracts notice. In this large clinical study, the alternative psychological treatments, one cognitive and the other interpersonal, are being pitted against each other and against antidepressant drugs (Waskow et al., 1979).

My general thesis is that it is important for us to understand that such clinical trials are simply <u>one</u> manifestation of a new direction rather than <u>the</u> new direction. If we review recent history regarding theory and research, this point will become more clear. We appear to have come to the end of an era in outcome research. It was introduced by H. J. Eysenck's publication in 1952 of "The Effects of Psychotherapy" (Eysenck, 1952), in which he concluded from a search of the literature that the effects of psychotherapy are "small or nonexistent." Moreover, he questioned whether psychotherapy produces significant positive change over everyday events in a person's life.

Eysenck's devastating critique was responded to by a preoccupation with the question of whether psychotherapy was a useful response to psychologically induced sources of human pain and misery. By psychologically induced, I refer of course to those vicissitudes that are invited or exacerbated by a person's own ways of thinking, feeling, or acting. As psychotherapists, we are particularly concerned with the way people contribute to the effects of their personal and impersonal environment. Since the early 1960s a vast amount of research has been devoted to the "bedrock" question of whether psychotherapy has any effect on the human condition. With time and attention, the sophistication of research designs has grown tremendously and the oversimplification of the original question has been fully delineated. Finally, we progressed to an ever more comprehensive and precise synopsis of the import of these accumulating investigations. Contributions to this process have been made by L. Luborsky (Luborsky et al., 1975), J. E. Meltzoff and M. Kornreich (1970), Allen E. Bergin and M. J. Lambert (1978), M. L. Smith and G. V. Glass (1977), and M. L. Smith, G. V. Glass, and T. I. Miller (1980), and although a few dissenters remain, the consensus is that research has demonstrated a sound basis for believing that psychotherapy does have a significant impact on the way a person lives his or her life.

Thus, we have ceased to challenge the authenticity of psychotherapy as an enterprise. In a sense that challenge was always more restricted than it seemed. So long as no challenge to the authenticity of human psychological misery can be made, then psychotherapy can be seen as an intrinsically worthwhile effort to deal with it, ignorance and ineffectuality notwithstanding. Our response to our ineffectiveness in the treatment of cancer has simply been to redouble our efforts, not to abandon them. So should this be our response with regard to the treatment of psychological problems. We must get on with the job of defining and validating forms of treatment for particular kinds of problems.

To do this job we must be able to study the interactions between human problems and treatments. The collaborative study of the treatment of depression represents an example of the clinical testing of two psychological treatments that have been specifically designed to apply to this particular psychological condition. While clinical trials of this sort are a necessary part of the sequence of research on psychotherapy, there are pitfalls in this part of the sequence, and it should be viewed as a limited part of a larger whole.

First, take note of the further elements revealed by the accumulating summaries of evaluative research. Although these summaries have assured us of the significance of the results attributable to psychotherapy, they have been much less definitive when it comes to evaluating different traditions of treatment, either overall or as applied to a particular condition. Except with regard to the treatment of phobias by behavioral methods, the various treatments are not markedly differentiated either in general or with regard to specific conditions. These statements, of course, apply only to the universe of investigations that qualified for inclusion in these reviews. There are many treatments and treatment targets that have not been represented in the research literature by formal investigations or by the kinds of controlled investigations and sound research designs that warrant their inclusion.

CLINICAL TRIALS

The demonstrated significant effects of psychotherapy are modest enough to tell us that there is need for much greater knowledge in order to attain greater precision in treatment. Because of this, it seems clear that our further research energies should be directed toward that goal. Clinical trials are important as a kind of concluding step in such a search. They may also serve an initial exploratory purpose.

My fear is that in clinical trials we may be deluded by analogy to the use of drugs as a treatment. We may act as though we already know the nature of the treatments we are studying. Even the most structured treatments do not come very close to capturing all of the events that accompany an encounter of any significant duration between two people. Any time two or more people meet and interact, we have an event that could be examined at many levels with attention to a variety of modes of expression. There are the manifest and the latent elements in the multiple patterns of communication. There is a range of attention from gross to fine detail. I am referring to the differences between intended effects and inadvertent ones, to the differences in socially demanded expressions of attitude that might be conveyed by the content of verbal expression or gross physical movements, or by the nuances conveyed subtleties of intonation patterns, and fine physical movements or postures. As the duration of the relationship increases, the opportunities for uncontrolled and unspecified elements in the treatment multiply.

Those who have sought to specify and structure treatments have not been unmindful of this problem. There is growing interest in developing treatment manuals. Yet even the best of these fall far short of the needed control (see G. Klerman et al., 1979). For the most part they give figural status to small parts of the total aspects of the interactional events. Moreover, virtually all of the present treatments are not homogenous processes. They are more accurately described as a grouping of actions "packaged as a treatment." To increase the effectiveness of treatment, we must first obtain the kind of knowledge which permits us to sift through that package to separate those portions that are needed to effect change from those whose function is merely superfluous.

If my description of the state of affairs is accurate, then it follows that we cannot afford to take such specified treatments and the clinical trials too seriously. More thorough analysis and hence more precise information, will allow us to identify the aspects of our treatment encounters that are mere rituals designed to satisfy the therapist, as differentiated from the aspects of the encounters that are truly instrumental in facilitating or effecting change.

I have not been close to the collaborative projects on depression. From my distance, it appeared that the original design did not include provisions for getting behind and beyond the treatment manuals. Eventually, provision was made for some analysis in that direction. Since I do not know the details, I do not know whether the additional analysis will only go behind the manual, that is, whether it will determine which specified actions and events are implicated in the change process. Going beyond the manual requires efforts to examine that part of the interaction that might be ground from the point of view of the developers of the treatment, but might be figural from other treatment developers' points of view. This latter step would be illustrative of the initial exploratory purpose of good clinical trials.

A major purpose of clinical trials is to establish an empirical bridge, which is necessary whenever we abstract and develop constructs to account for the phenomena that have aroused our curiosity. The usual processes of science carry us from these stripped down formulations to stripped down conditions of observation, during which we seek to test the tenability of these formulations. Having stripped the original source of our curiosity down to its hypothetical essentials and tested our hypothesis under the specially controlled conditions that permit that test, we are ready to return to the original source of our curiosity. The philosopher of science, F. S. C. Northrup (1947), has referred to this as the obtaining of epistemic correlation, which "joins a thing known in one way to what is in some sense that same thing known in a different way." Thus the clinical trial functions as a final step that assures us that the abstracting and simplifying process that marks scientific methodology has not, through oversimplification, led us into an engrossing blind alley. An abstracted treatment model, validated under laboratory conditions with pseudopatients, may not in fact bring about the same results in clinical trials with actual patients. This suggests that the process of simplification has left out some important factors in the events that were the original targets of our curiosity.

I summarize my argument by stating that the present and future task of research on psychotherapy is to get behind treatment-change target interactions to gain the knowledge that will provide greater power for change. This means getting inside treatment packages. It means forming a conceptual structure that allows us to understand the differences and similarities across treatments and their consequences.

THEORY AND RESEARCH

A growing number of us have become convinced that the theoretical model of the therapeutic working alliance offers a heuristically rich base for assimilating known data and promises a bountiful harvest of new data. Most importantly, it speaks to the psychotherapist in a manner that facilitates the improvement of his or her work.

Practitioners and researchers alike have come to the rueful conclusion that psychotherapy research has had little or no impact on practice. There have been two reasons for this. First, past research has been obsessively preoccupied with the more general question of whether existing treatments were of any value. It offered little compelling evidence that would force a choice among methods. Second, as T. S. Kuhn (1962) has pointed out with regard to scientific theories, changes occur when a new paradigm is adopted. I offer the therapeutic working alliance model as a candidate for such a new paradigm.

Since these terms were first introduced by psychoanalytic theorists, it would be best to start with the question of whether this is in fact a new theory or an imperialistic effort to bring all treatment under the psychoanalytic umbrella. Parenthetically, Aaron T. Beck (e.g., 1976), using the terms "collaborative empiricism," has applied a similar concept to his cognitive treatment. A distinction is made between the strength of the working alliance and the type of working alliance. Following the psychoanalytic prescriptions leads to one kind of working alliance. Following other treatment theories can lead to different kinds of alliances. I will develop the thesis that the client and patient tasks associated with these prescriptions are a key part of the differences in types of therapeutic working alliances.

Briefly, these terms refer to the partnership that develops when a person offers herself or himself as the agent of change. The strength of that partnership resides in the degree of agreement that is achieved regarding the change goals and the methods or tasks that will be instrumental. An effective component, called "bonds," enters into the partnership to the degree that these bonds are inevitable results of the shared activities and that these bonds facilitate the carrying out of the tasks of the alliance. Observation and reflection suggest that the conditions of virtually all therapeutic partnerships create and require bonds of trust (possibly the most crucial) and liking and caring.

There are at least three discernible stages in a therapeutic alliance: (1) the initial information or contract; (2) the period of work; and (3) the period of completion and dissolution.

In earlier formulations, I had offered the proposition that the amount of change achieved in a particular working alliance was a function of the strength of that alliance, which resided in the fullness of agreement with regard to goals, tasks, and the appropriateness of the bonds. If the strength of the alliance is a major factor in change, and if two or more traditions of treatment experience the same range of success in achieving strong working alliances, these traditions would not be expected to differ in effectiveness. This is a formulation that could account for what we have observed about different treatments. They all have their various successes and failures, which make it difficult to establish differences in success rates. If we were to concentrate on understanding the obstacles toward achieving strong alliances within each tradition and gain knowledge that would bring alliances within control, this would surely lead to an increase in success rates or, where the obstacles are insurmountable, to decreasing the amount of wasted effort.

Further elaboration has led to a distinction between the strength of the alliance at the end of the initial stage of formation and the strength of the alliance through the working stage (see Bordin, 1980). The strength of the alliance at the end of this initial stage, often referred to as the "elementary working alliance," is not yet assumed to be the maximum that will characterize the successful partnership. But it must be strong enough to endure the strains of hard work in the partnership. The harder the work to be engaged in, the stronger this elementary alliance will need to be. Moreover, the time and effort needed to secure the required elementary working alliance may vary considerably as a function of the psychological condition and situationally influenced state. For example, an extremely time consuming effort is required to build an elementary alliance in the therapy of both borderline and schizophrenic patients. In the case of borderline patients, the barrier to be overcome in order to form an elementary alliance is the tendency to use the relationship as an end rather than for change. With schizophrenic patients, mistrust of self and the other must be overcome. In both instances, the most arduous and most modifying part of the treatment is represented in that initial phase.

Whatever the required strength of the elementary working alliance, the work of the partnership in the middle phase has a strengthening effect, assuming that the change agent is skillful and the work progresses. One of the inevitable effects of such a shared experience is the strengthening and deepening of a bond. But the work usually is accompanied and facilitated by further clarifications of goals and by experiencing the relevance of tasks as a means of achieving those goals. The general trend during a successful treatment will be toward increasing strength in the alliance. This will be an undulating trend, marking momentary set-backs in the face of difficulties experienced by the patient in carrying out his or her tasks, due to the effects of the very personal characteristics in which his or her psychological problems reside. The work of surmounting this strain on their partnership represents work on the very characteristics that brought the patient to seek psychotherapy in the first place. The appropriately selected therapeutic task has helped to create a laboratory in which therapist and patient can experience, examine, and learn how to modify the patient's problematic ways of thinking, feeling, and acting.

I believe that we have here the basis for a new paradigm to guide future research on psychotherapy, directed toward taking apart the package of goals and tasks embedded in various treatment modalities and gaining the knowledge about the therapeutic power of various tasks. This will give us the basis for constructing new and more powerful, as well as more precisely aimed, packages. Apart from the work on instrumentation of measures of strength[1] and on developing taxonomies of goals and tasks accompanied by discriminating procedures, the implementation of this research paradigm calls for a series of steps. These steps are:

1. Confirmation that the strength of the working alliance can account for the amount of change, independent of the kind of working alliance;
2. Examination of the process of building and repairing working alliances; and
3. Study of the power and interchangeability of various therapeutic tasks as a means of bringing about change.

After some comments on instrumentation, I will elaborate on each of these steps. With regard to measuring the strength of the working alliance, it is important that all three aspects be examined, including goals, tasks, and bonds. Measures based especially on patient report, and to some degree on therapist report, run the danger of reflecting mainly the bonding aspects. Moreover, unless these reports are based on the initial period, they are likely to be increasingly contaminated with the outcome and at the same time reflective of undulations in the strength of the alliance during the middle period.

If we are to study the process of building and repair, very finely grained measures are needed. Retrospective reports would not appear to be good bets for achieving this latter goal. After refining what we mean by a goal of psychological treatment, the development of a taxonomy would seem to require construction of a specificity-generality dimension. As suggested earlier, I generally define the goal of psychological treatment as a change in the way a person reacts to his or her environment, particularly to other people or impersonal conditions, which are usually the targets of social and political movements. One could elect to try to modify the external conditions, which is environmental manipulation and is also the target of social and political movements. In the psychotherapeutic enterprise we are concerned with the individual's complicity in what happens to her or him. In different approaches to psychotherapy I can discern differences, usually theoretical, in various change targets, and this plays a part in the specificity or generality of the change that is implicitly or explicitly negotiated during the period of alliance formation.

I consider it highly likely that the kind of thinking that has gone into the various diagnostic manuals will interact with an evolving taxonomy of therapeutic tasks. Although I have been principally interested in those tasks that enter into the partnership constructing phase, it is possible that the varieties of working alliances will not be very distinguishable in terms of alliance building tasks; their differences appear in their goals and in middle task involvements.

Although not completely unequivocal, encouraging evidence has begun to accumulate regarding the relevance of the strength of the working alliance as a forecaster of either disaffection from therapy or degree of success (Luborsky, 1976; Sarnat, 1975). A recent satisfaction study carried out in L. S. Greenberg's group at the University of British Columbia adhered most closely to my theoretical specifications regarding the measurement of strength. The investigator, A. O. Horvath (1981), found a substantial correlation between the strength of the working alliance and outcome across a heterogeneous sample of therapies. The types of therapies represented included cognitive and behavioral, client-centered, Gestalt, and humanistic. The sample was not large enough to permit analysis by type of therapy. I understand that replications are being pursued, which may permit further analyses of the accumulated data.

Thus, there are good beginnings with this phase of research. While the British Columbia group included all aspects of the working alliance in their measurements, they relied on reports by therapists and patients (separate measures), taken at that point in therapy when an elementary alliance had been developed. There remains the question of how this form of measurement would fit in with the observations by third parties such as that which has been obtained by the groups from the University of Pennsylvania, Vanderbilt University, and the University of Michigan.

If the building and repair of working alliances were demonstrated as important sources of change, developing a fuller understanding of those processes would enable us to augment our therapeutic power. A recently completed study by E. Lansford (1982) at Michigan represents a beginning at developing a system of observation of the repair process and an initial demonstration that sensitivity to weakening in the alliance and effectiveness in repairing those breaks is correlated in the expected direction with outcome. Earlier at Michigan, S. A. Lehrke (1978) had explored systems of observation designed to identify the modes of interaction that facilitate the development of a strong working alliance. As an example of this, a therapist's failure to respond except by listening to a patient's expressions of interest or concern regarding alliance-related matters is predictive of alliance failure.

These are only beginnings. In the long run we need systematic studies of the vicissitudes of building strong partnerships within the various traditions of therapy to assure ourselves that the principles of alliance building are general for all kinds of alliances or require modifications according to the type of alliance. Moreover, we need empirical tests of the generality of the assumption that the tasks embedded in various therapies all contribute to the change process by tapping into the patient's problematic reactions. Of course, one likely outcome is that engaging in the task sets in motion a change process independent of the role of self-imposed obstacles.

This brings us to research on the tasks, especially those of the middle phase of collaborative work. If we guard against over simplification and over generalization, certain elements of the behavioral approach are potentially fruitful. I am referring to the effort to arrive at a precise proposition that will enable us to identify exceptions to our belief, and to investigate them in simplified situations more amenable to control, manipulation, and replication. Specifically, I am advocating a strategy by which we identify therapeutic tasks and subject them to examination. Many elements of such an approach have been represented in the research on systematic desensitization. In doing this, we open the possibility of bringing together many diverse strands of knowledge drawn from general theories and research. A key task in desensitization is for the patient to imagine himself or herself engaged in a series of actions. (J. L. Singer, 1974; see also Horowitz, 1983, who are taking off from the European strand of theory and research on imagery, and have stimulated expanded and renewed research interest.)

In addition to observing the impact on a person of engaging in a particular task, we must examine how the characteristics of the person influence his or her engagement and the impact it has. The work of E. T. Gendlin (1968) on the client-centered task of experiencing comes to mind as an example. We must not lose sight of the fact that these are collaborative tasks, which means that the change-agent participates in them. Our concern with impact and individual differences must include the therapist. Specifically, this includes what it is that the task requires of her or him, what effect it has on her or him, and what personal characteristics may make it difficult to do his or her part. I think it promises to provide the answers sought by the voluminous research on A and B psychotherapists.

Research on the task can provide a basis for controlling the profusion of therapies. By selecting key tasks for this kind of examination, we can not only test the validity of their underlying assumptions but identify redundancies in tasks. Let me illustrate with regard to the two tasks of free association, which is so central to psychoanalysis: the task of experiencing, emphasized by client-centered therapy, and imaging, featured in desensitization. B. Weitzman (1967) reported his observation that free association seemed to be embedded in the process of imaging as it occurred in a desensitization process. Lansford and I (1983) had an opportunity to study the overlap between ratings of free association and experiencing. Using some analogue data collected earlier in a study of individual differences in the response to the task of free association, we rated the same response on the Experiencing Scale and found evidence of considerable overlap.

The results of such research should go beyond a simple winnowing of treatments. This research has the potential to lead to broader understandings of the elements in therapeutic tasks, their critical therapeutic power, and the surrounding conditions that permit that power to be exercised. This is, of course, the dream of glory and power that keeps researchers on psychotherapy going, and it is the social justification for the expenditures of energy and resources.

NOTES

1. A great amount of work has already been done. (See, for example, D. E. Hartley, 1978; A. O. Horvath, 1981; L. Luborsky, 1976; E. Marziali et al., 1981; and E. R. Ryan, 1973.) More up-to-date summaries of the above cited and later relevant research are to be found in the work of L. S. Greenberg and W. M. Pinsoff (1986).

REFERENCES

Beck, A. T. 1976. Cognitive Therapy and the Emotional Disorders. New York: International Universities Press.

Bergin, A. E. and M. J. Lambert. 1978. "The Evaluation of Therapeutic Outcomes." In S. L. Garfield and A. E. Bergin, eds. Handbook of Psychotherapy and Behavior Change. 2nd ed. New York: Wiley.

Bordin, E. S. 1980. "Of Human Ties that Bind Free." Presidential address, meeting of Society for Research in Psychotherapy, Pacific Grove, California.

Eysenck, H. J. 1952. "The Effects of Psychotherapy." Journal of Consulting Psychology 16: 319-24.

Gendlin, E. T. 1968. "Focusing Ability in Psychotherapy, Personality, and Creativity." In J. M. Shlien, ed. Research in Psychotherapy. Vol. 3. Washington, D. C.: American Psychological Association.

Greenberg, L. S. , and W. M. Pinsoff, eds. 1986. The Psychotherapeutic Process: A Research Handbook. New York: Guilford.

Hartley, D. E. 1978. "Therapeutic Alliance and Success in Brief Individual Therapy." Ph.D. diss. Vanderbilt University.

Horowitz, M. J. 1983. Image Formation and Psychotherapy. New York: Jason Aronson.

Horvath, A. O. 1981. "An Exploratory Study of the Working Alliance: Its measurement and Relationship to Therapy Outcome." Ph.D. diss.

University of British Columbia.

Kuhn, T. S. 1962. The Structure of Scientific Revolutions. Chicago: University of Chicago Press.

Lansford, E. 1982. "Weakening and Repairs of the Working Alliance in Short-Term Psychotherapy." Ph.D. diss. University of Michigan.

Lansford, E., and E. S. Bordin. 1983. "A Research Note on the Relation between Free Association and Experiencing Scales." Journal of Consulting and Clinical Psychology 51: 367-69.

Lehrke, S. A. 1978. "Working Alliance Development Early in Psychotherapy." Ph.D. diss. University of Florida.

Luborsky, L. 1976. "Helping Alliances in Psychotherapy: The Groundwork for a Study of Their Relationships to its Outcome." In J. L. Claghorn, ed. Successful Psychotherapy. New York: Bruner/Mazel.

Luborsky, L., B. Singer, and L. Luborsky. 1975. "Comparative Studies of Psychotherapies: Is It True that 'Everyone Has Won and All Must Have Prizes'?" Archives of General Psychiatry 32: 995-1008.

Marziali, E., C. Marmar, and J. Krupnick. 1981. "Therapeutic Alliance Scales: Development and Relationship to Psychotherapy Outcome." American Journal of Psychiatry 138: 361-64.

Meltzoff, J. E., and M. Kornreich. 1970. Research in Psychotherapy. New York: Atherton.

Northrup, F. S. C. 1947. The Logic of the Sciences and the Humanities. New York: Macmillan.

Ryan, E. R. 1973. "The Capacity of the Patient to Enter an Elementary Therapeutic Relationship in the Initial Psychotherapy Interview." Ph.D. diss. University of Michigan.

Shapiro, D. A., and D. Shapiro. 1982. "Meta-Analysis of Comparative Therapy Outcome Studies: A Replication and Refinement." Psychological Bulletin 92: 581-604.

Sarnat, J. E. 1975. "A Comparison of Psychoanalytic and Client-Centered Measures of Initial In-Therapy Patient Participation." Ph.D. diss. University of Michigan.

Singer, J. L. 1974. Imagery and Daydreams: Methods in Psychotherapy and Behavior Modification. New York: Academic Press.

Smith, M. L., and G. V. Glass. 1977. "Meta-Analysis of Psychotherapy Outcome Studies." American Psychologist 32: 752-60.

Smith, M. L., G. V. Glass, and T. I. Miller. 1980. The Benefits of Psychotherapy. Baltimore:

Johns Hopkins University Press.

Waskow, I. E., S. Hadley, M. B. Parloff, and J. Autry. 1979. Unpublished manuscript. Clinical Research Branch, National Institute of Mental Health, Rockville, Md., March.

Weitzman, B. 1967. "Behavior Therapy and Psychotherapy." Psychological Review 74: 300-17.

13

Using Videotape for Supervision, Training, and Research

Lynn Simek-Downing

This introduction to the use of videotape as a training, supervisory, and research instrument will illustrate the interactive aspects of this important medium. In my training of psychotherapists, counselors, medical students, and residents, the most valuable training tool I have found, next to the professor's interactions, is the videotape. Let us first examine the role of the supervisor, then basic training modalities using videotape exercises and feedback, and lastly examine the uses of videotape in research.

SUPERVISION AND TRAINING

The professor who trains students in psychotherapy is the first supervisor of future clinicians' work. The professor teaches the skills, approaches, and theories that he or she believes are the most important, thereby transmitting his or her worldview. The professor also shares his or her personal therapeutic work through case discussions and illustrations of successful interventions. By using this modeling approach to "good" psychotherapy, he or she engages the students in a relationship of molding or training. As the instruction continues, supervision is more overt, through commenting on students' work in practice exercises, through cassette tape recordings, or through videotapes of the students with simulated or real clients. This initial supervision enormously influences the students' future performance, attitudes, behaviors, values, and professional ethics in the practice of psychotherapy. The word "supervisor," as used henceforth, will mean one who trains and supervises the initial professional work of students of psychotherapy, one who gives training and process comments on professional client/therapist relationships to psychologists and psychotherapists working in the field.

The role of the supervisor is multifold, including the roles of teacher, psychotherapist to the student, formulator of ethical standards, and processor. The cornerstone of successful supervising is the establishment of a strong, open, and honest relationship with each supervisee. The process of relationship establishment can be enhanced by the use of constructive comments, by allowing mistakes and by using these for learning, by discussing alternatives, using awkward moments for growth, by using oneself as an example in formulating professional ethics and work habits, and by modeling open and honest communication.

Although the components of establishing a sound supervisory relationship are generally the same, the methods of supervision vary widely, from oral reporting, to the one-way mirror, to various types of recording. Oral reportage of a counseling interview has only been shown to be 50 percent effective, and clients report different items of importance than do therapists. Cassette recordings of counseling and psychotherapy sessions omit the vital information of eye contact and body language. The superiority of videotape recordings is due to its inclusive ability to completely repeat the session, reporting information on eye contact, body language, and vocal tone and rate. One can have an instant replay of a particular moment and can stop, discuss, and review the session at any interval. Additionally, the videotape can be saved and reviewed for working on particular issues over time and for charting progress.

Although the videotape provides a superior replication of a psychotherapeutic session, there are some inherent drawbacks. First, the equipment is expensive to purchase and maintain and may not be available or feasible for private practitioners. It also takes a much longer period of time to review a videotape, due to the fund of information provided by the recording. A supervisee cannot always videotape every client, due to time, facility, or refusal of clients to grant permission, and therefore a selection of one or two recordings may not be indicative of the overall performance of the student in psychotherapy. Some new research indicates that both the client and the student counselor feel awkward during a videotape session and that, therefore, may inhibit the client/therapist interactions and relationship. With all these disclaimers, videotape can still be most effective when used as a primary tool for supervision, even if used sporadically, and when used in combination with other methods of supervision.

Any examination of a videotape application must first give an overview of a complimentary training model. Training and teaching models vary almost as widely as individual differences among professors, and much research has been generated on which model is the "best."

There are three factors that are always at play in the psychotherapy process: the client, the psychotherapist, and their relationship. In the role of educator or supervisor, the same three factors are in interplay, but experienced as the supervisor/teacher, the supervisee/student, and their relationship. The client or student has his or her own worldview and ways of defining the world, as well as personal spheres of influence--including social, personal, familial, economic, racial, environmental, cultural, religious, physical, and so on. Also, each client or student is at a unique stage of development in his or her life cycle and has inherent developmental goals. Likewise, the psychotherapist or teacher has his or her own worldview, spheres of influence, and developmental issues. The interplay of these two people engaged in an intimate relationship is the context of psychotherapy whether the stage of the psychotherapy is a private practice, a community mental health center, or a prison. The engaging of the client in the process of psychotherapy, or the student in supervision, is the initial stage of psychotherapy or teaching and can be viewed as the "trust return rate" or groundwork for the entire future of the relationship. Not every therapeutic approach is applicable to every client; neither is every educational approach pertinent to every student. Rather, it becomes a part of the diagnostic procedure to assess what therapy is appropriate for which time, and what educational approach will work the best with which student.

The distinct advantage of the use of videotape in the process of both psychotherapy and education is that it is essentially an objective observer of the process. It does not carry any inherent values and can be used by people of any theoretical persuasion or any training modality. Since the commencement of recording interaction of social significance on film (J. Collier, 1969), many suggestions have been made about the efficiency and efficacy of using visual recordings (A. Summerfield, 1983; P. Ekman and W. Friesen, 1978). Other researchers and teachers have developed specific skills and training programs that are widely in use across the continents (A. Ivey, 1971, 1978; N. Kagan et al., 1968). Still other researchers and teachers have made specific applications and investigations across a vast range of the psychotherapeutic process including nonverbal behavior (R. Harper et al., 1978), social behavior and family therapy (M. Berger, 1978), teacher education (F. Fuller and B. Manning, 1973), and virtually any other application you may consider, being far too many to include here. The point stands that there is a universal creativity and applicability to the use of videotape for supervision and training that can incorporate any system of values, approach to psychotherapy, or educational curriculum.

RESEARCH APPLICATIONS

Although there is a plethora of literature on the application of videotape to the process of psychotherapy and education, not nearly as much has been generated on the research applications of videotape. Some early studies used the application of the videotape to specific skills or sequences within a given psychotherapeutic or educational modality such as self-confrontation (Fuller and Manning, 1973; Ivey, 1978), or feedback (Kysilka and Anderson, 1972). The use of videotape in teaching individual counseling skills, or microcounseling, and evaluating the learning process was reviewed by Allen Ivey and Jerry Authier (1978).

The clinical and educational applications of videotape are quite global, as it is used for review, processing, discussion, stimulation, and overall training and development. Conversely, the research applications of the videotape are very specific including a frame-by-frame or individual interactional examination of the communication process (Simek-Downing and Quirk, 1985; Simek-Downing et al., 1986). Rating systems have been devised (Ash and Sattler, 1973) that have a high inter-rater reliability and wide applications beyond the research setting (Backman, 1979). The videotape is desirable for a research tool because it can be reviewed by many raters, can be saved and reviewed as many times as desired, can be reversed, and has a freeze frame. For those who are used to using a one-way mirror or hand recording social interactions, the advent of videotape in the research arena is truly revolutionary.

One of the questions frequently posed by those who engage in video-based research is the one of how contaminating the use of videotape is to the result of the research. Particularly of concern is the effect of the videotaping on the participant and the participant's reactivity. Some of the considerations of the changes that might occur in research due to participant reactivity to the videotaping are outlined by C. Renne, P. Dowrick, and G. Wasek (1983) and include the following four factors:

1. increases or decreases in rate of behaviors;
2. increases or decreases in the magnitude, severity or duration of behaviors;
3. appearance of behaviors that interfere with the intentions of the study; and
4. the introduction of new, unrepresentative responses.

There are no definitive answers to this question, and research on the applications of client and participant reactivity to videotaping have found both positive and negative findings. The negative effects of the videotaping were found in feeling uncomfortable (Carmichael, 1966) or inhibited (Gelso, 1972), client dissatisfaction (Gelso, 1973), and inhibited self-expression (Tanney & Gelso, 1972). Other research findings show no adverse participant reaction on self-disclosure in group therapy (Stempf, 1977), in the psychotherapeutic relationship (Kagan et al., 1950), or adaptation to the performance situation (Purcell and Brady, 1965). Most of the researchers feel that the use of videotape has an initial contamination effect while the participant is adjusting to the environment but that, after the initial trepidations are over, the videotaping is forgotten and the machine is not a negative variable. Much of the anxiety the participant may feel in being videotaped can be overcome if the issue is treated sensitively and properly at the time of engaging the participant in the research project, by talking about the uncomfortable feelings and by being direct at the time of receiving consent.

As an illustration of how videotape can be used

for research, I would like to present a research project that applied a line-by-line analysis of communication skills used by medical students (Simek-Downing and Quirk, 1985).

This research project investigates medical students' interviewing skills before and after a six-week clerkship in family and community medicine. Male and female medical students participating in a clerkship in family and community medicine were asked to conduct pre- and post-videotape interviews with a simulated patient. After the pre-test videotape, the student received feedback from the simulated patient and from a faculty member. Students then participated in a six-week clerkship with a family physician. Multivariate and univariate analyses of variance of pre- and post-test interviews showed significant pre-post differences on seven of ten interviewing skills and focal areas. Significant differences relating to the students' year in medical school were also found.

METHODOLOGY

Fifty randomly chosen third and fourth year medical students, 25 males and 25 females, were asked to conduct a patient interview that was videotaped at the beginning of a six-week clerkship in family and community medicine. Simulated and real patients presented standard problems that included headaches, stomachaches, and back pain.

The faculty member, student, and patient reviewed the videotape, stopping after certain segments for discussion and feedback. Areas for discussion and feedback included opening the interview; discovering the reason for the visit; questioning techniques; maintaining focus; using empathy and reassurance; using paraphrase and summarization; vocal tone, volume, and rate; body posture and eye contact; vocabulary; and closing the interview.

Teaching students how to open an interview included asking them to shake hands, introduce themselves, explain their role, ask the patient what he or she would like to be called, and using the patient's name. Discovering the reason for the visit included teaching the student to ask an open question and to realize that the reason for the visit may or may not be the same as the chief complaint. Teaching of questioning techniques stressed beginning with open questions and moving to more specific questions. Teaching how to maintain focus included staying on the topic, providing transitions between topics, and balancing the interview to include the following: the areas of chief complaint, psychosocial, personal, and family medical histories; and a review of the systems pertinent to the chief complaint. Teaching students how to use empathy and reassurance focused on how students can offer feelings, support, and reassurance in an empathic manner. Teaching how to use paraphrase and summarization included teaching how to provide a transition to a new topic, how to involve the patient in the summary, and how to summarize at the closing of the interview. Students were also taught appropriate vocal volume, tone, and speech rate. Feedback was given to students regarding body postures, with an emphasis on comfort and attentiveness. Feedback was given to students on their eye contact, with the goal of having it be observant, consistent, and varied with feeling. Students were taught to use the patient's own words, explain medical terms, avoid medical jargon, ask the patient if he or she understands the medical terms, and engage in patient education. Finally, the students were taught to close the interview by providing a summary, a transition to the physical exam, an opportunity for final questions and/or disclosures, a follow-up visit, and if necessary, a referral.

Following the tutorial, the students then spent the remainder of their six-week clerkship practicing these skills in an ambulatory setting with a family physician. After completion of the six-week clerkship, students were again asked to make a videotape with a simulated patient.

Each statement in the pre-test and post-test videotape interviews was analyzed for interviewing skills, focus, and nonverbal language. Interviewing skills included open questions, closed questions, paraphrase, summarization, patient education, eliciting feelings, interpretation, and characterization of factors such as location, duration, and quality.

Open questions are those that need explanation and cannot be answered in one word. Closed questions can be answered in one word, usually yes or no. Paraphrase is the reiteration of a few of the patient's words in the context of a physician's statement. A summary includes a synopsis of the thoughts, feelings, and issues that have been most important in the preceding discussion. Patient education includes the disseminating of information to or training of the patient. Eliciting feelings refers to any action on the part of the physician to understand, discover, or label the patient's feelings. Interpretation refers to the relabeling or redefining of a patient's thought, feeling, or action from the physician's viewpoint. Focal dimensions included chief complaint, past personal and family medical history, psychosocial history, and systems review.

Each student received a weighted score for each skill and focal area, based on the proportion of responses related to that category. Multivariate and univariate analyses of variance with repeated measures were used to compare pre- and post-test scores, in relation to the independent variables of sex of the student and year of training.

RESULTS

The findings revealed that of the three independent variables assessed, year of medical school, sex of the student, and clerkship experience, the latter was the most influential on focal content and verbal interviewing skills. Independent of year of training and sex, students exhibited differences on seven of the ten skills and focal areas assessed before, as compared to after, their core clerkship experience.

With reference to focal content area the students increased the number of responses directed to the chief complaint and decreased the number of responses related to psychosocial and past personal and family medical history.

For verbal skills, students increased their use of summaries and patient education, but decreased the number of paraphrases and open questions.

The focal area that appeared to be influenced by all the variables studied was systems review.

Overall, fourth-year students asked more questions related to systems review than did third-year students. The results also indicate that fourth-year students showed a greater decrease in questioning related to systems review than did third-year students. Finally, women showed a greater decrease over time in the number of questions related to systems review.

DISCUSSION

The marked increase in responses asking information about the chief complaint may be due to the educational variable of the videotaped intervention, the preceptor's training, and/or the students' experiences during the clerkship. This increase can be compared with the decreases in responses seeking information about psychosocial issues and past personal and family medical history. This seems to show a trend toward more focus on the presenting problem and less emphasis on viewing other aspects of the patient's life, that is, historic and personal milieus.

One possible explanation for this finding may be that students don't observe their busy preceptors engaging in this type of interviewing. This is supported by the findings of such authors as P. Byrne and B. Long, (1978) who concluded, after observing over 2,000 doctor-patient interactions, that most of the general practitioners they had observed were unable or unwilling to enter into any real relationship with patients. In this connection they state:

> This is made very apparent by the way in which these doctors prevent and stifle any expression of feeling in the consultation. Throughout the interviews there is an apparent desire to maintain their relationships with patients almost on a technocratic basis. One may even suspect that these very impersonal styles are defense mechanisms which protect doctors against patients (p.117).

Another explanation is that there are fewer opportunities than expected in the office setting for students to observe and practice comprehensive interviewing. This may be the result of the continuous nature of the relationship between family physicians and their patients. The psychosocial ingredients of the relationships vis à vis the interviewing techniques necessary to establish them may not always be evident to the student who spends only five or six weeks in the physician's office. If either of these explanations is viable, then we, as educators and role models for future family physicians, should discuss how we can better train students to view patients in a Gestalt or holistic perspective.

Students used more summaries and provided more

patient education. By contrast, they used significantly fewer open questions and paraphrases. The trend here seems to be away from patient-centered skills (open question and paraphrases) and toward physician-centered skills (directives, patient education, and summarizing). Students seem to be focusing more quickly on a diagnosis, with less exploration of other aspects of the patient's life or symptoms. This may be due to an increasing medical data base and may reflect an increased mastery of knowledge of internal systems. Conversely, it may reflect the development of medical "tunnel vision" that perpetuates the role of physician as director of the interview and detracts from fostering an appropriate physician-patient relationship. Byrne and Long observed a distinct preference by the physicians they observed to deal with the first "organic" complaint registered by the patient. These physicians failed to follow up on psychosocial issues raised by the patient. In addition, these physicians tended to investigate the organic aspects of illness using closed questions that were likely to elicit yes or no responses from the patient. Again, this brings to the forefront the questions such as "What is it that we want to teach about interviewing to future family physicians?" and "What is the best method of teaching this to students?".

The only significant overall effect of a year in medical school was in relation to review of systems. Most of this may be attributable to the fact that all fourth-year students have had their medicine rotation, during which systems review is stressed as an interviewing focus. During the family medicine clerkship, the emphasis on systems review is variable, according to individual preceptors. Overall, one would expect more limited review based upon the relevant systems. It is therefore encouraging that fourth-year students, who have gained greater mastery of the systems review, also showed greater decline in the number of statements related to this area.

The results of this research may provide evidence of trends in contemporary medical education such as most emphasis being placed on diagnosis and treatment of the "organic" presenting problem. While this is always necessary, it should neither preclude the importance of treating the patient within a systems approach nor work at the expense of providing a conducive physician-patient relationship to augment the healing process. One could conclude that current training in family medicine should use a more integrated teaching approach, including training in investigating psychosocial and past personal and family medical histories as well as chief complaint. Also, family physicians who teach medical students should realize the importance and impact of their roles in the modeling of future family physicians.

Although this research project has focused on communication skills with aspiring physicians, the basic videotape research techniques could be applied to students of counseling, psychotherapy, clinical psychology, education, or human sciences.

CONCLUSION

The use of the modality of videotape is an essentially value free objective tool that can be of value to those who are engaged in the training of psychotherapists or other helpers. The benefits of using the videotape are far more influential than the inherent drawbacks. The research possibilities for the use of videotape in all social and psychological settings have only begun to be explored. With the portability of the new camcorders, the use of the videotape, now a common household item, opens numerous new avenues for the exploration in both education and research. The possibilities seem almost limitless, and the disadvantages seem to dwindle with familiarity. The videotape provides the educator, supervisor, or researcher with a readily available, flexible, portable, and diversified tool that awaits the creativity of the user.

REFERENCES

Ash, M., and H. Sattler, 1973. "A Videotape Technique for Assessing Behavioral Correlates of Academic Performance." Research in Education, 8, no. 8: 62-63.

Backman, C. 1979. "Epilogue: A New Paradigm?" In G. Ginsburg, ed. Emerging Strategies in Social Psychology Research. Wiley: New York.

Berger, M., ed. 1978. Videotape Techniques in Psychiatric Training and Treatment. New York: Brunnel/Mazel.

Byrne, P., and B. Long 1978. Doctors Talking to Patients. London: Her Majesty's Stationery Office.

Carmichael, H. 1966. "Sound-Film Recording of

Psychoanalytic Therapy." In L. Gottschalk, and A. Overbach, eds. Research Methods in Psychotherapy. New York: Appleton-Century-Croft.

Casswell, S. 1983. "Applications of Recording Human Performance." In P. Dowrick and S. Biggs, Using Video. New York Wiley.

Collier, J. 1969. Visual Anthropology. New York: Holt, Rinehart, Winston.

Ekman, P., and W. Freisen. 1978. Facial Action Coding System. Consulting Psychologists Press.

Farmer, J. 1971. "Indigenous, Interfactional Research." Resources in Education 6, no. 9: 135.

Fuller, F., and B. Manning. 1973. "Self Confrontation Reviewed: A Conceptualization for Video Playback in Teacher Education." Review of Educational Research 43, no. 4: 469-528.

Gelso, C. 1973. "Effect of Audio-Recording and Videotaping on Client Satisfaction and Self-Expression." Journal of Consulting and Clinical Psychology 40: 455-61.

Gelso, C. 1972. "Inhibition Due to Recording and Client's Evaluation of Counseling." Psychological Reports 31: 675-77.

Harper, R., A. Wiens, and J. D. Matarazzo. 1978. Nonverbal Communication: The State of the Art. New York: Wiley.

Ivey, A., and J. Authier. 1971, 1978. Micro-Counseling. Springfield, Ill: Charles Thomas.

Kagan, L. 1969. "The Electrical Recording of Social Casework Interviews." Journal of Nervous and Mental Disease 148: 365-74.

Kagan, N., P. Schauble, and D. Resnikoff, "Interpersonal Process Recall." Social Casework 31: 371-78.

Kysilka, M., and B. Anderson. 1972. "A Study to Evaluate Supervisory Feedback for Student Teachers." In ERIC Educational Documents Abstracts New York: MacMillian Information.

Purcell, K., and K. Brady, 1965. "Adaptation to the Invasion of Privacy: Monitoring Behavior with a Miniature Radio Transmitter". Merrill Palmer Quarterly 12: 242-54.

Renne, C., P. Dowrick, and G. Wasek. 1983. "Conditions of the Participant in Video Recording." In P. Dowrick, and S. Biggs, eds. Using Video. New York: Wiley.

Simek-Downing, L., and M. Quirk. 1985. "Videotape Analyses of Medical Students' Interviewing Skills." Family Medicine 17, no. 2, (March-April, 1985): 57-60.

Simek-Downing, L., M. Quirk, and D. Letendre. 1986. "Simulated Versus Actual Patients in Teaching Medical Interviewing." Family Medicine 18, no. 6 (November-December 1986): pp. 358-60.

Stempf, C. 1977. "The Effects of the Presence of Video-Recording on Self-Disclosure in a Group Therapy Setting as a Function of Repression and Sensitization Defensive Styles." Dissertation Abstracts 37: 5380.

Summerfield, A. 1983. "Recording Social Interaction." In P. Dowrick, and S. Biggs, eds. Using Video. New York: Wiley.

Tanney, M., and C. Gelso, 1972. "Effect of Recording on Clients." Journal of Counseling Psychology 19: 349-50.

Persons Name Index

Subject Index

About the Contributors

DIANE B. ARNKOFF is Associate Professor in the Department of Psychology at the Catholic University of America. She is the author of numerous articles and chapters on cognitive therapy, psychotherapy integration, cognitive assessment, and social-evaluative anxiety. She is currently a member of the steering committee of the Society for the Exploration of Psychotherapy Integration.

ALLEN E. BERGIN is a professor of psychology at Brigham Young University (1972 to present) and former Director of the Values and Human Behavior Institute there (1976-78). He was previously professor of clinical psychology at Teachers College, Columbia University (1961-72). He is a fellow of the American Psychological Association, past president of the Society for Psychotherapy Research (an international organization), past president of the Association of Mormon Counselors and Psychotherapists, and a member of the Society for the Scientific Study of Religion. He is a diplomate in clinical psychology of the American Board of Professional Psychology and is on the Professional Board of the American Mental Health Foundation.

He has served on the editorial boards of ten professional journals and has been a consultant to the National Institute of Mental Health and the Peace Corps. He edited the Handbook of Psychotherapy and Behavior Change (with Sol L. Garfield) and coauthored Changing Frontiers in the Science of Psychotherapy (with Hans H. Strupp). He has published 60 articles and books, and his papers have been reprinted in two dozen anthologies. Two of his publications (with Garfield and Strupp) have been named Citation Classics by the Institute for Scientific Information.

He was educated at the Massachusetts Institute of Technology, Reed College, Brigham Young University (B.S., 1956; M.S., 1957), Stanford University (Ph.D., 1960, Albert Bandura, Advisor), and the University of Wisconsin (postdoctoral fellow, Carl R. Rogers, Advisor). He has been a visiting professor at the University of Minnesota and University of Utah and has delivered more than 200 lectures at universities and conferences in the United States and eight other countries.

He has held community service positions in the areas of human resources, mental health, education, family life, and religion in New Jersey, New York, California, and Utah. He and his wife Marian are the parents of nine children.

His current professional interests include personality theory and research; values, religion, and mental health; and evaluation of psychotherapy.

MARK H. BICKHARD has a B.S. in mathematics, an M.S. in statistics, and a Ph.D. in human development, with a specialization in clinical psychology, all from the University of Chicago. He is currently professor of educational psychology at the University of Texas in Austin and has a private practice in psychotherapy. Previous works include _Cognition, Convention, and Communication_ and _On the Nature of Representation_ (with D. Michael Richie), and _Knowing Levels and Developmental Stages_ (with Robert L. Campbell). His interests focus on the nature and origins of psychological processes. The theory that has emerged from these interests is generally known as _interactivism_, a term derived from a core characteristic of the theory's basic epistemology. A major current emphasis is the development of the interactivist model with respect to issues in personality, psychopathology, and psychotherapy.

EDWARD S. BORDIN is the Professor Emeritus of Psychology at the University of Michigan in Ann Arbor. He is the author of many journal articles and books, including _Psychological Counseling_ (1955, 1968) and _Research Strategies in Psychotherapy_ (1973). He has received the Career Award from the Division of Counseling Psychology, American

Psychological Association, and the Career Research Award from the Society for Psychotherapy Research.

MARYANNE GALVIN is a licensed psychologist who uses hypnotherapy in her private practice in Boston, MA. She has held faculty positions at the University of Massachusetts, Amherst; Mt. Holyoke College; the University of New Hampshire; Northeastern University; Wheelock College; and Tufts University School of Medicine. Dr. Galvin has received travel research awards for psychological investigations in South America from the National Science Foundation and a private foundation sponsoring scholarly activity in the USSR. Her interest and dedication to cross-cultural psychology and psychotherapy outcome and training research is demonstrated by her many publications in these fields. Dr. Galvin holds the Diplomate in Counseling Psychology from ABPP, National Register Membership, and fellowships in the Massachusetts Psychological Association and the American Psychological Association.

SOL GARFIELD has had a varied career as a clinical psychologist since receiving his Ph.D. from Northwestern University in 1942. He served as a clinical psychologist in the U.S. Army in World War II and in several hospitals and clinics of the Veterans Administration. He has also been very much involved in training other clinical psychologists, as the former director of training at three university clinical psychology programs and as director of psychology at a medical school.

For over 40 years Dr. Garfield has been involved in practice, teaching, and research in the area of psychotherapy. In particular, he has been interested in the proliferation of therapeutic approaches, the importance of potential common factors in psychotherapy, and the evaluation of outcome in psychotherapy. Dr. Garfield is a former president of the Division of Clinical Psychology of APA and of the Society for Psychotherapy Research.

NICK HEATHER was born in London, England, in 1938 and obtained a B.A. (Hons.) in psychology from the University College, London in 1965. After various occupations in psychology, he received a M.Sc. in clinical psychology from the University of Leeds in 1971. He worked as a clinical psychologist in the British National Health Service until 1978, when he turned to full-time research in addictive behaviors. He founded the Addictive Behaviors Research Group at the University of Dundee and has recently taken up a post as Professor of Drug and Alcohol Studies and Director of the National Center for Drug Research at the University of South Wales, Sydney, Australia. He is the author of seven books and over fifty publications in scientific journals.

G. MARIAN KINGET is a native of Belgium, where she obtained her Ph.D. cum laude from the University of Louvain in 1948. Soon thereafter she enrolled at Columbia University as a foreign Ph.D postgraduate, and she published her dissertation as The Drawing Completion Test in 1952. Life Magazine published a three page illustrated article on it on June 9, 1952.

In 1950 she left Columbia for the University of Chicago, where she worked directly with Carl R. Rogers for two years. At the request of the University of Louvain, she wrote a book introducing the Rogers approach to the European community. Psychotherapie et Relations Humaines (two volumes) which was translated into four other languages.

Since 1952, she has taught at Michigan State University and remained in contact with Rogers, her coauthor for Volume 1 of the foreign publications and continues to create new courses, write and speak. Her latest book, On Being Human, was reprinted in 1987, both as a text book and a trade book. She is now a citizen of the United States.

MICHEL LEGRAND is a professor at the Catholic University of Louvain and university Faculty, N.D., of the Paix à Namur (Belgium). He works in the domains of epistemology of psychology, social psychopathology and community psychiatry, and institutional analysis. He is author of many volumes and articles including Rapports de pouvoir, famille et technologies psychologiques, Louvain-La-Nueve: Cabay, 1983; Psychanalyse, Science, Société, Brussels: Mardaga, 1984; and La psychiatrie alternative itelienne entre mythe et réalité, Toulouse: Privat, 1988.

MICHAEL J. MAHONEY received his Ph. D. from Stanford University and is now Professor of Counseling Psychology at the University of California at Santa Barbara. The author of 12 books and numerous scientific articles, Dr. Mahoney helped pioneer the "cognitive revolution" in psychology and is a continuing contributor to the growing interface between the cognitive and clinical sciences. Honored as a fellow by the American Psychological Association, he was chosen to be a Master Lecturer on Psychotherapy Process in 1981. Dr. Mahoney has received several professional awards, including a Fulbright Award in 1984, the Faculty Scholar Medal from Pennsylvania State University in 1982, and a 1985 Citation Classic from Science Citation Index in recognition of the influence of his 1974 book Cognition and Behavior Modification.

Dr. Mahoney has served on the editorial boards of 12 scientific journals and has worked with the U.S. Olympic Committee since 1978 in the area of sport psychology. His research interests include basic processes in psychological development, cognitive theories and therapies, psychology of science, and health and support psychology. His forthcoming book, Human Change Processes: Notes on the Facilitation of Personal Development, attempts to integrate the research literatures from several disciplines as they bear on the conceptualization and facilitation of psychological change.

AUGUSTO PEREZ GOMEZ is a professor of psychology, at the University of the Andes, Bogotá, Colombia. He teaches psychopathology, research strategies in psychotherapy, and treatment strategies for drug addicts. His current publications are "Cocaine and basuco: an overview of Colombia, 1985," in The Cocaine Crisis (New York: Plenum, 1987); Cocaina: nacimiento y evolución de un mito (Bogota: Catalogo Cientifico, 1987), "La Re-interpretation du phenomene psychotherapeutique, Psychotherapies (Geneva, in press); "Der Gebrauch von Kokain: Einige bemerkungen zu seiner Auswirkung und Behandlung," forthcoming; and, Historia de la drogadicción en Colombia (Bogotá: Tercer Mundo, in press). At present, he is the director of La Casa, a program for drug addicts. He is also working as a consultant to the United Nations program in Colombia, in the field of evaluation and research.

LYNN SIMEK-DOWNING is an Associate Professor of Family and Community Medicine at the University of Massachusetts Medical Center, where she trains medical students and family practice residents in communication skills, medical interviewing, community medicine, family systems, and family medicine, as well as supervises the Worcester Health Care for the Homeless Project. She is also a psychotherapist in private practice. She received her B.A. in psychology from Clark University and her Ed.D. in counseling psychology from the University of Massachusetts, Amherst. She developed her interest in cross-cultural issues in psychotherapy from her interest in anthropology and her desire to train counselors and psychotherapists. While studying and teaching at the University of Massachusetts, Amherst, she wrote Counseling and Psychotherapy: Skills, Theories and Practice with Allen Ivey, now in its second edition. This work stresses her commitment to training and developing culturally appropriate counselors and psychotherapists.

HANS H. STRUPP received his Ph.D. from George Washington University in 1954 and has been a member of the faculty at Vanderbilt University since 1966. He holds the position of Distinguished Professor of Psychology. Before coming to Vanderbilt, he was on the faculty of the University of North Carolina at Chapel Hill. Dr. Strupp has been engaged in psychotherapy research for 35 years and has published extensively on this topic.

PAUL WACHTEL is a Distinguished Professor of Psychology at City College, New York, and the Graduate Center of the City University of New York. He received his undergraduate degree from Columbia University and his Ph.D. from Yale University. He is also a graduate of the Postdoctoral Program in Psychoanalysis and Psychotherapy at New York University. He is the author of Psychoanalysis and Behavior Therapy (1977); The Poverty of Affluence: A Psychological Portrait of the American Way of Life (1983); Family Dynamics in Individual Psychotherapy (1986); and Action and Insight (1987), and is editor of Resistance: Psychodynamic and Behavioral Approaches (1982).

www.ingramcontent.com/pod-product-compliance
Ingram Content Group UK Ltd.
Pitfield, Milton Keynes, MK11 3LW, UK
UKHW020800290926
15470UKWH00003B/874

9 780275 930967